Praise for FAT IS NOT YOUR FATE

"Drawing on research from the Human Genome Project, the nutritionist authors help readers identify their own particular genetic programming or phenotype . . . and provide eating plans tailored to each one. Its recipes and healthy food lists are good, and it includes an outstanding portion-control system."

—*Library Journal*

"Dietitians Mitchell and Christie dispel the notion that your weight is necessarily hostage to your genes. Instead, they look at six types of people prone to weight gain and offer a diet tailored to each. The authors recommend physical activity and frequent small meals consisting of protein and carbohydrate food as a healthy alternative."

—Bev Bennett, AP

"Dr. Mitchell and Dr. Christie have done it again. They've taken a new and complex nutrition and diet related topic, thoroughly researched it, and interpreted it so that readers can understand it and easily take action to improve their health."

— Ellen T. Carroll, M.S., R.D., Senior Editor/Food Development Director, *Cooking Light*

"Two of Florida's most respected members are the first to address this progressive approach to weight loss. Christie and Mitchell offer successful eating plans based on the latest genetic research in this fascinating book."

—Christine Stapell, Executive Director, Florida Dietetic Association

What some of Susan's and Cathy's clients are saying about their weight-loss plan:

"Losing weight was easier than I thought. What worked for me was knowing what to do and having a simple plan. Now I don't just grab whatever's quick and easy. With the Phenotype D plan, I've been able to eat things I like and still lose weight."

—CL, Florida

"I was tired of being heavy and tired of people saying stuff to me. It's a mental thing . . . how you look at yourself. What you look like is how you feel, and I didn't feel good about either. The Phenotype C diet plan changed the story of my life. I could never have lost 100+ pounds without it. Before, I lived to eat; now I eat to live."

—JB, Florida

"My success has exceeded my expectations. I'm a Phenotype D and so far I've lost 23 pounds. No diet has done this for me before. I think about what I'm doing now. I shop differently. I didn't want another fad diet—I wanted a lifestyle change. I don't count calories or measure anything *and* I don't feel deprived ever. That's the key for me."

—Linda K.

"I had to throw away my pants and buy new ones. I've dropped two pant sizes and lost 15 pounds. Now I have more energy and brain power plus I've saved a lot of money because I quit eating junk. My blood work has improved. This Phenotype E diet is awesome!"

—John L.

FAT IS NOT

YOUR FATE

Outsmart Your Genes
and Lose the Weight Forever

Susan Mitchell, Ph.D., R.D., FADA and
Catherine Christie, Ph.D., R.D., FADA

A Fireside Book
PUBLISHED BY SIMON & SCHUSTER
New York   London   Toronto   Sydney

FIRESIDE
Rockefeller Center
1230 Avenue of the Americas
New York, NY 10020

This Fireside Edition 2006

FIRESIDE and colophon are registered trademarks
of Simon & Schuster, Inc.

For information regarding special discounts for bulk purchases,
please contact Simon & Schuster Special Sales at
1-800-456-6798 or business@simonandschuster.com

Designed by Katy Riegel

Manufactured in the United States of America

10   9   8   7   6   5   4   3   2   1

Library of Congress Cataloging-in-Publication Data
Mitchell, Susan, Ph.D.
    Fat is not your fate : outsmart your genes and lose the weight forever /
Susan Mitchell, Catherine Christie.
        p.   cm.
    Includes bibliographical references and index.
    1. Weight loss.   2. Phenotype.   I. Christie, Catherine.   II. Title.
RM222.2.M5438   2005
613.2'5—dc22   2004052247

ISBN-13: 978-0-7432-5039-9
ISBN-10:   0-7432-5039-7
ISBN-13: 978-0-7432-4986-7 (Pbk)
ISBN-10:   0-7432-4986-0 (Pbk)

Most of the individuals described in this book are composites,
and names and other characteristics have been changed.

To my husband, Charlie,
who encourages me to let my dreams
take flight and cheers me
along each step of the way. I love you.
　　　　　　　　　—Susan

To my husband, Leo.
I love waking up with you
each morning and look forward
to coming home
to you every night.
　　　　　　　　—Catherine

Acknowledgments

To our agent, Julie Castiglia: Your business savvy, insight, and advice are priceless. We truly appreciate your support and commitment to our work and to us.

To our editor, Caroline Sutton: Thank you for seeing the vision of this book. Your attention to detail, experience, dedication to the project and creativity have been invaluable. Working with you and Simon & Schuster is an honor and a pleasure.

To the family and friends who share our excitement for this book, thank you for your unending love, support and input:

Dudley, Nancy, Matt, Emily and Molly Mitchell; Dotty and Al Olsen and the Olsen family; Ellen Griffin; John Soper; Tim Tew; Deanna Tompkins; The Livera family; Linda Neuman; Jane Dennis, R.D.; Emmy Haigler; Dr. Linda King; Jerry Bingham; The Cards of Card's Opticians; Julia Lynn Picarello, R.N.

Ben Wilcox, Barbie Ryals, Virginia Wilcox; Tara, Norman, Kalyn, and Trentin Spears; Theresa Christie; Sue and Buzz Crane; Jan and Ron Szalkowski; Karen Christie and Ed Hughes; Jo Shuford Law and Richard Law; Dan and Sylvia Schultz; Patty Thomas and Fred Fletcher; Carolyn and Bill Rayboun; Claire Lorbeer, Alice Rhatigan, Vilma Willard, Brenda Keen; Lori Valencic; Toni Martin; Rosemary Jacobs, Nita Bell; Judy Perkin; Judy Rodriguez; Simin Vaghefi; and Sally Weerts.

Special thanks to: Tershia d'Elgin for her expertise in editing and writing; Becky Johnson, MFA, Laura Kittleson, and Virginia Braddock, M.S.,

R.D., for their help early on in reading, editing, and commenting on the manuscript. And to Gail Bentzon for artwork; Marlene Stiwalt; Dorine Smith, R.D.; Ellen T. Carroll, M.S., R.D.; Kay Braddock; Linda Kamus; Dr. Eli Porth; Dr. Zulma Cintron; and Dr. Andrew Giles.

Contents

Foreword

Many of us want to know the best way to lose weight and keep it off. Since I began practice as a registered dietitian, I have seen diets come and go. Everywhere you look, you can find testimonial success stories from diets so wildly different it seems impossible. Claims for everything from high-protein/low-carbohydrate, high-carbohydrate/low-fat, or no-exercise-needed, to eat grapefruits only, live on raw food, or drink vinegar every day. Nutrition knowledge and recommendations do change but they should change based on the latest science. Perhaps it is a testament to the importance of nutrition that such a vast amount of research is being done in this area.

Fat Is Not Your Fate offers a bold new way to look at the weight loss issue. Dietitians understand the importance of individualizing diet advice to get optimal results. One diet definitely does not fit all. Looking at genetics through family history, these authors have used the latest research to fine-tune simple, easy-to-follow, individualized diets. The weight comes off, stays off, and you improve your health at the same time.

I congratulate these authors, both of them registered dietitians and active members of the American Dietetic Association, for writing a book that asks the question Is overweight due to genetics or environment? and answers that question honestly—it's both. In order to lose weight, both genetics and environment are key. Through the Phenotype Assessment, you can determine your genetic health risks and follow the diet best suited for you to lose weight and improve or protect your health. Through the

Weight Trigger Quiz, you will examine your personal routine, find what contributes to your weight problems, and then follow recommendations for changing those issues specific to you. This is what makes this book unique!

This is a journey to make each of us as healthy as we can be. Please join me in discovering your own phenotype and environmental risk factors that affect us individually.

Here's to your health!

Marianne Smith Edge, M.S., R.D., L.D., FADA
MSE & Associates, LLC
President, American Dietetic Association (2003–2004)

CHAPTER 1

Outsmarting Your
Genetic Legacy

WHY A PHENOTYPE-BASED DIET?
THE LINK BETWEEN GENETICS AND WEIGHT

Though weight problems may be hereditary, they need not be a life-long affliction. Our experience as nutrition professionals upholds this, and emerging genomic data demonstrates why. You can stop thinking of your genes as a curse. This book will show how your genes can work for you, instead of against you. The right foods in the right proportions with the right supplements, tied specifically to your genetic profile, will produce genetic equilibrium and the weight loss you want. Within days, you will feel healthier and more satiated. This weight loss can work, for a lifetime, because the diet is exactly tailored to your body and health concerns, as portrayed in the physical expression of your DNA called your *phenotype*.

The logic behind our new individualized phenotypal approach is evident in a truism that anyone who has ever dieted knows firsthand—that the diet that works great for some people is for others an exercise in futility. Diets are almost as diverse as people—low-calorie diets, high-protein diets, low-fat diets, grapefruit diets, cabbage soup diets, vinegar diets . . . the list goes on and on. Diet effectiveness is inconsistent because the dietary chemicals within food act at a molecular level on specific genes, and no two people's genes are the same. Added to the problem of not knowing which diet will work for you is the fact that most trendy diets are unhealthy. Even if they result in weight loss, they work against long-term well-being and may actually do irreversible damage, especially as dieters keep trying new ones to counteract recurring weight gain.

The good news is that the uncertainty is over and that these unhealthy diets are no longer necessary! With the help of science, we can now characterize more than ever before the molecular activity of dietary chemicals. We can explain why diets don't come in one-size-fits-all. This has taken the guesswork out of dieting and revolutionized weight loss. It has also made weight loss far more healthy.

Unlike gimmick dieting, gene-based nutrition diminishes the likelihood of weight-related maladies such as high blood pressure, diabetes, and cardiovascular disease. In fact, this program is entirely unique because it provides an individualized diet, guaranteed to succeed, that will alleviate the weight-related malady to which you're most vulnerable. You'll lose weight and feel better on a phenotype diet because the foods are compatible with you, on a cellular level.

Even though our program is structured around micromechanisms, you needn't visit a clinic or register for a program. You needn't spend a lot of money on gene profiling. Everyone can match him- or herself to one of our diets right away, using this book as a guide.

We have confidence in your ability to make the most of your genetic inheritance, because this program has helped hundreds of our patients and clients synchronize their foods and eating habits with their genes. Consistently, good health and weight loss flowed from their efforts. One patient, a cardiologist who had just been diagnosed with type 2 diabetes, came to us because she was not getting results from the high-carbohydrate, heart-healthy diet recommended at the time. Whenever she ate a plateful of pasta, her blood sugar rocketed. A glucose receptor problem related to her genes and extra weight barricaded her cells against blood sugar. Glucose accumulated in her bloodstream. We knew she needed a diet personalized to her genetic risk for diabetes, not the general recommendation. A lower-total-carb diet, combined with high-fiber carbohydrates and protein, worked better. When we customized her diet, she lost weight and kept it off.

In another example, an overweight and hypertensive police officer couldn't meet his department's rigorous fitness requirements. With his excess weight and high blood pressure, this client was a heart attack waiting to happen as he rolled through the city on his motorcycle. He needed a personalized diet to tame his sodium-sensitive genes into directing the hormones that control blood pressure more effectively. We loaded his cycle saddlebags with dried fruit and restricted his trips to sodium-loaded fast-food joints. He lost weight and decreased his blood pressure.

The secret to both these patients' successes wasn't the diet trend of the week. It was in their genes.

GENE DISCOVERIES REVOLUTIONIZE DIETING

For more than ten years, we developed individualized dieting programs like these, based on empirical evidence. At the same time, researchers were striving to understand the genetic basis of weight. Then, in 1994, a Rockefeller University team, under Dr. Jeffrey M. Friedman, identified the first "obesity gene." The discovery of one of the obesity genes shouldn't have been so amazing, since everyone had always taken the hereditary nature of obesity for granted. But in a popular, trend-driven field such as weight control, it was a watershed for researchers and practitioners alike.

If science could explain how obesity occurred, it might also explain how to undo it. That was the hope. Researchers continue to move between models and microscopes, hastening to expose other obesity genes. Concurrent with the well-publicized race to create a comprehensive Human Genome Map, the Human Obesity Genome Map was launched at the 1994 International Congress on Obesity, using research from all over the world. In it, data from published reviews is extensively cross-referenced, then linked to databanks internationally. Scientists found, importantly, that specific genes or gene mutations mismanage the body's ability to utilize nutrients, including protein, fats, and carbohydrates. Over seventy genes are now on the Human Obesity Genome Map. Tellingly, common obesity genome sequences often contain genes that increase the likelihood of disease. Only infrequently do mutations in one gene cause trouble. More often, illness and weight problems stem from complex interactions between numerous genes and other stimuli. This fact mirrored conditions we had witnessed in our patients and clients.

Optimistic about the ramifications of the burgeoning obesity genome, a growing number of people are jumping on a revolutionary new bandwagon called nutritional genomics or "nutrigenomics." The University of California at Davis is leading the way with its new Center of Excellence for Nutritional Genomics. Duke University is partnering with the Center for the Advancement of Genomics on the Genomic-Based Prospective Medicine Project to develop a truly modern and individual-based form of healthcare. The European Union has launched NuGO, a network for integrating this new branch of research.

Like most scientists, nutritional scientists had always turned to nature and nurture for explanation. Nutrigenomics connects nature and nurture, putting them on the same two-way street. Just as nature (i.e., genes) affects nurture (i.e., environmental influences such as foods, stress, and habits), nurture also affects nature. Nutrigenomics shows that nutrition can actually alter an individual's "nature," i.e., their genetic expression.

Nutrigenomic scientists scrutinize this nature–nurture interaction through a fine lens. Doctors and dietitians continue to assess concentrations of nutrients found in the urine, blood, and body tissue. With the help of technology, scientists are beginning to ascertain the actual molecules that food contains and how cells use those molecules to maintain or disrupt well being. As an example, naturally occurring phytochemicals such as the flavonoids in red grapes and berries slow the onset of heart disease. In another example of nutrigenomic research in practice, people with an explicit genetic profile may have a risk of heart disease due to the high levels of amino acid homocysteine. Increasing the B vitamin, folate, in their diet diminishes homocysteine in their blood. Foods high in antioxidants, such as fresh produce, protect the cells' ability to function normally, which is particularly important for diabetics and people with metabolic syndrome. These examples are germane because heart disease and diabetes often accompany weight problems.

In sum, *we are what our genes tell us to be* and *we are what we eat, too,* right down to the distinct chemical constituents of any given food product. The interface is nutrigenomics, a field almost unknown as recently as five years ago. In the future, the nutrition-gene link will use data from personalized gene testing to assemble even more personalized food prescriptions for health.

Inexpensive, applicable gene profiling is still years off, but our practice was already changing people's lives with diets based on their specific relationship of family history (i.e., genetics), weight, and diet. Immediately, incontrovertible scientific evidence of the hereditary character of weight problems validated the approach we had developed over the years. It verified the logic of our applied nutrition techniques, right down to their impact on individual receptors on cell surfaces. Our methodology, we learned, was based on phenotypes.

THE PHENOTYPE FACTOR

Being clear about what a gene is and what it isn't will help explain phenotypes. A gene is a recipe for making a protein. Our very lives depend on these proteins because they precipitate each and every physiological action at a molecular level. However, each gene just sits there, as though in a recipe box, unless it is activated. For its particular protein to get made, a gene has to be turned on, or *expressed,* by a trigger. These triggers are chemical, a confluence of interactions first among genes, and second between genes and added elements like food and stress. The chemicals bind to receptors on the cell surface, then a trigger goes off and the protein is produced. The gene is expressed, doing what it was designed to do.

Genes that are expressed result in physical manifestations called *phenotypes.* (*Pheno* is from the Greek word for "shining.") Thus, genotype is what your genes are, the fifty-fifty inheritance from your mother and father's contributions; phenotype governs what you shine like, or look like, and determines your predisposition to health as well as to specific diseases. Only the expressed genes—usually a whole linkage of expressed genes—matter (except in relationship to passing the genes on to one's offspring that might express them). Only they result in a phenotype.

How do genes turn on and turn off? And at what point? Research suggests that expression begins in utero, influenced by the mother's habits, eating and otherwise. After birth, the chemical triggers are either induced from outside the body (as from eating, breathing, or absorption through the skin) or from inside the body (as when emotions precipitate an infusion of hormones). The whys and wherefores of phenotypes are still poorly understood.

As is so often true, the explanation is evident in the exceptions. Research indicates that children of overweight parents aren't necessarily doomed to stoutness, even as embryos. The proof of this is in small-size people whose DNA contains obesity genes. Even carrying around, cell by cell, a genetic arsenal of fat-fate tendencies, the gun never goes off. According to the emerging understanding of the way genes work, that is because, for one reason or another, their obesity genes were not *expressed,* or activated. These exceptions seem to prove that genetic destiny is not immutable. If everyone whose genome holds obesity genes isn't fat, then clearly phenotype manipulation is the answer.

We knew this from our practice, not from people who weren't overweight, but from people who were. From years in the weight loss trenches, we had accumulated all kinds of proof that diet influences the messages delivered to the brain. Take, for example, people who reach for carbs during times of stress. Genetically, they usually have low levels of serotonin, which increase the risk for depression and overeating. Stress produces a release of the hormone cortisol, which triggers their desire for carbohydrate. The carbohydrates then catalyze reactions that increase serotonin production, sending soothing messages to the brain. Unfortunately, the excess calories this generates tend to accumulate at the waist.

Altering the amount and type of food our patients and clients consumed, and when they consumed it, delivered dietary chemicals to cells in ways that let them lose weight instead. Following custom diet plans, they became thinner and healthier, with different eating impulses and improved satiety. According to the science, they were altering their genetic expression, manipulating their phenotype by changing their habits and food choices to facilitate explicit chemical reactions.

Here is how dietary chemicals work. Not everything we swallow gets metabolized for fuel or storage. For example, vitamins, minerals, and phytochemicals are not stored or used for fuel but are highly involved in controlling metabolic processes. Some dietary chemicals, called *ligands*, peel off and bind to proteins, effectively "turning on" certain genes. When diets are out of balance, genes that would be better unexpressed light up. This might change carbohydrate metabolism or increase blood pressure. It might elevate blood glucose or increase blood homocysteine levels or any number of other bad effects. Alternatively, eating conscientiously limits damage to the cells and protects their ability to function normally. Importantly, as everyone's genetic mix differs slightly in composition, people react differently to the same ligands. Two people, even two related people, will not necessarily react to dietary chemicals the same way. One person's balanced diet is another person's increasing pants size. Clearly, therefore, one key to optimizing genetic equilibrium is personalized nutrition.

DNA-BASED WEIGHT LOSS THAT WORKS

As we said, we had always accepted that some diets worked for some people and not for others. Each client or patient completed our assessment before treatment, and its outcomes then shaped the individualized nutritional prescription. As we started looking at our cases, and reading the emerging data on nutrigenomics, we realized that we were phenotyping people with these assessments. And the specific nutritional programs we designed for these phenotypal patients and clients were the last and only diet they'd ever need.

The phenotypes provide a shortcut to genotyping, because they can be profiled easily and inexpensively. Again, this means that gene-based nutritional programs are not just for the future, and not just for people who can afford gene profiling. We knew people could outwit their genetic destiny, because our patients were doing it. Our approach already included specific tools for converting problematic phenotypes into mechanisms for weight loss. However, what was needed was an effective strategy to help, not just people who came to us directly, but swaths of people with essentially the same problems.

Grouping the data according to parallels, six distinct phenotype categories—each associated with unwanted weight gain—became apparent. These are as follows:

Six Weight Gain Phenotype Categories

Phenotype A: Addiction-linked weight gain
Phenotype B: High blood pressure–linked weight gain
Phenotype C: Cardiovascular disease–linked weight gain
Phenotype D: Diabetes-linked weight gain

Phenotype E: Emotional eating–linked weight gain
Phenotype H: Hormone-linked weight gain

People in these six groups share a very similar genetic destiny. Just as the research indicated, these weight gain–causing phenotypes also correlate with disease-causing conditions—addiction, high blood pressure, cardiovascular problems, diabetes, emotional eating, and hormone imbalance.

Our objective was to design six weight loss regimes, matched to the six phenotypes, with the right balances of nutrients that *feel* satisfying because they *are* satisfying. First we developed assessments to help people determine their predominant phenotype, then carved out six diets to guide them toward weight loss and better health. We will explore the diets in detail in subsequent chapters.

We began systemizing, testing, and refining the approach. Client after client, class after class, people asked us to tell them what to eat, how much to eat and when to eat it. Before suggesting regimes, we presented the latest nutrition research. We asked questions. We asked them to fill out our assessments. The clients and patients investigated which of the six phenotype programs applied to them specifically. Feeling empowered to buck their genetic fate, they made changes in their diets and environments.

A client named Tamara was a case in point. She was an emotional-eating virtuoso, alternating between deprivation and indulgence. Her husband regularly accused her of "cheating" on her various diets. His hurtful comments sabotaged her weight loss, made her feel deprived, and actually increased the emotional eating, part of what characterized her as a Phenotype E. Hers was a clear pattern of revenge eating. After five weeks of following the Phenotype E Diet, she lost 12 pounds and gained more energy plus felt like she had control over her eating.

Jay, 5'8" and 260 pounds, was barely 30 years old when he had a liver transplant. His poor eating and exercise habits were not only keeping him from losing weight; they had compromised his liver and blood lipids, particularly cholesterol. Clearly, something had to give. After six months on the Phenotype C Diet, Jay had dropped a total of 50 pounds. It's been more than five years and Jay is still following the diet. He's taken 100 pounds off, and, more importantly, he's kept it off.

Specific diets worked on a molecular level to modify these people's genes and their phenotypal expression. *Tamara and Jay were leaner and healthier within two weeks.* Similarly, one of these six diets will bring you the weight loss you seek. Because you are on the right diet for you genetically, you will feel better, look better and have more energy. It will also work preventively to minimize the diseases historically associated with your weight problems.

Moreover, the right foods that contain beneficial dietary chemicals reduce the influx of problem ligands that have been turning on your disease-causing, weight gain–causing genes. Potentially and by contrast, they will also encourage the expression of genes that will optimize your health, longevity, and well-being. In this manner, phenotype dieting *actually changes who you are.* It's as easy as first determining your genetic and personal risks through our assessment and quiz, then following the regime designed for that phenotype. *Your genes define you—they should define your diet.*

CHAPTER 2

Learn Your Phenotype and What Triggers Your Weight Gain

The Phenotype Assessment and the Weight Trigger Quiz

Consider the adage "The apple never falls far from the tree." Your family tree contains your genetic health history. Its less desirable fruits may include obesity. They may include addiction, high blood pressure, depression, heart disease, diabetes, or any of the approximately three thousand genetically derived illnesses. However, that your roots produced a few rotten apples need not spoil your future. This is because "nature" is only part of the phenotype story. You have almost complete control over the other part, "nurture," particularly if armed with the up-to-date scientific background we're about to give you.

This chapter is your opportunity to take stock of your intrinsic genetic nature and evaluate your positive and negative weight triggers. Taking the Phenotype Assessment will identify your phenotype, which is the manifestation of the genes you are presently activating. Taking the Weight Trigger Quiz will identify destructive habits that may be working against a thinner and fitter destiny. Together, the results of these assessments will help you make best use of the coming chapter on your particular phenotype.

YOU ARE THE EXPERT ON YOU

In many ways, no one knows more about your genome than you do. The infinitesimal chains of DNA of which you are made, though invisible, impart a dense history, which you can "read" and analyze whenever you wish.

We designed our Phenotype Assessment to help you interpret what you know about yourself.

The assessment demonstrates that weight gain is never an isolated problem. A propensity for weight gain, in a family and in an individual, is almost always associated with other health difficulties, as we've said. In fact, obesity may soon overtake smoking as the leading cause of *preventable* death, according to U.S. Surgeon General David Satcher, entirely because of its relatedness to other diseases. We do not treat weight problems in isolation from other aspects of our patients' and clients' lives, because to do so isn't healthy and because it doesn't make sense. Associated illness, or the anticipation of illness that comes from knowing family history, provides important background for distinguishing between the fat/fate phenotypes. Likewise, the related health problems point to the most effective treatment: the phenotype-personalized diets that make this book revolutionary.

The assessment is broken down into six phenotypes, each governed by common gene sequences. The first half of each phenotype concerns your heredity; the second half deals with your personal risk factors. The assessment asks you to consider your vertical lineage (parents and grandparents) as well as your horizontal lineage (sisters, brothers, aunts, and uncles). The more comprehensively you can trace your family's health history, the more informed you'll be about the medical conditions, cultural traditions, and social habits that affect your weight and health.

Please itemize what you know about your family, as well as yourself, honestly. Allow yourself time to think about your eating and behaviors in new ways. Talk to other family members about health and weight issues that may have affected them and previous generations. Your answers will identify your phenotype and direct you to your personalized weight loss program.

THE PHENOTYPE ASSESSMENT

Please read each statement under every phenotype and answer "yes" or "no" as it relates to you. If you don't know your family history or don't know the answer to a question, circle "DK" for Don't Know.

PHENOTYPE A

The genetic connection:

Y N DK   My mother has or had a substance abuse or addiction problem.

Y N DK   My father has or had a substance abuse or addiction problem.

Y   N   DK   One of my grandparents on my mother's side has or had a substance abuse or addiction problem.

Y   N   DK   One of my grandparents on my father's side has or had a substance abuse or addiction problem.

Y   N   DK   One or more of my siblings or half siblings has or had a substance abuse or addiction problem.

Y   N   DK   One or more of my blood-related aunts or uncles has or had a substance abuse or addiction problem.

My own risk factors:

Y   N   DK   I have been told by a physician or mental health professional that I have an addiction (substance/alcohol) or binge eating disorder.

Y   N   DK   I would describe one of my own behaviors as addictive.

Y   N   DK   My eating has become more compulsive after stopping the use of drugs or alcohol.

Y   N   DK   I gained significant weight after stopping the use of drugs or alcohol.

Y   N   DK   I have frequent cravings for salty, sweet, or fatty foods.

Y   N   DK   There are times when I feel that I cannot control what or how much I am eating.

Y   N   DK   I often eat alone because I feel embarrassed about how much I am eating.

Y   N   DK   After eating, I often feel depressed, disgusted, or guilty about overeating.

Y   N   DK   I binge-eat on an average of two days a week.

Y   N   DK   I consider myself to be a compulsive overeater/binge eater.

PHENOTYPE B

The genetic connection:

Y   N   DK   My mother has or had high blood pressure or a stroke.

Y   N   DK   My father has or had high blood pressure or a stroke.

Y N DK   One of my grandparents on my mother's side has or had high blood pressure or a stroke.

Y N DK   One of my grandparents on my father's side has or had high blood pressure or a stroke.

Y N DK   One or more of my siblings or half siblings has or had high blood pressure or a stroke.

Y N DK   One or more of my blood-related aunts or uncles has or had high blood pressure or a stroke.

My own risk factors:

Y N DK   I have been diagnosed with high blood pressure or hypertension.

Y N DK   My blood pressure typically runs **above** 120/80.

Y N DK   I am taking a blood pressure medication.

Y N DK   I drink more than 24 ounces of beer, 10 ounces of wine, or 2 ounces of liquor each day.

Y N DK   I am in a high-risk group for hypertension such as over age 60 or African-American.

Y N DK   I would describe myself as physically inactive.

Y N DK   I eat fewer than five fruit and/or vegetable servings a day.

Y N DK   I eat a diet high in processed foods or added salt or sodium.

Y N DK   I would describe my dairy product intake as rare or none.

Y N DK   I drink soft water (low in most minerals but high in sodium) rather than hard (high in minerals except sodium). In municipalities with hard tap water, some homes and businesses have water softeners installed. Bottled water brands vary greatly and can be soft or hard. If you are uncertain about tap water in your area, you can call your local water supplier for data.

PHENOTYPE C

The genetic connection:

Y N DK   My mother had a heart attack or was diagnosed with heart disease before age 65.

Y   N   DK   My father had a heart attack or was diagnosed with heart disease before age 55.

Y   N   DK   One of my grandparents on my mother's side has or had a heart attack or was diagnosed with heart disease.

Y   N   DK   One of my grandparents on my father's side has or had a heart attack or was diagnosed with heart disease.

Y   N   DK   One or more of my siblings or half siblings has or had a heart attack or was diagnosed with heart disease.

Y   N   DK   One or more of my blood-related aunts or uncles has or had a heart attack or was diagnosed with heart disease.

My own risk factors:

Y   N   DK   My bad (LDL) cholesterol level is **above** 100 mg/dl.

Y   N   DK   My good (HDL) cholesterol level is **below** 45 mg/dl (for men) or 55 mg/dl (for women).

Y   N   DK   I am taking a physician-recommended cholesterol-lowering drug or supplement.

Y   N   DK   I am a smoker or user of other tobacco products.

Y   N   DK   In addition to cholesterol concerns, I have high blood pressure.

Y   N   DK   I watch TV more than three hours a day or would describe my exercise level as inactive.

Y   N   DK   I would describe my intake of red wine and/or purple grape juice as rare or none.

Y   N   DK   I eat fast food more than twice a week.

Y   N   DK   In addition to cholesterol concerns, I have been diagnosed with diabetes.

Y   N   DK   I carry my excess weight predominantly around the waist as opposed to the hips.

PHENOTYPE D

The genetic connection:

Y   N   DK   My mother has or had diabetes or metabolic syndrome (three of the following symptoms: high triglycerides [**above** 150 mg/dl], waist measurement of **more than** 35 inches, blood pressure of **at least** 135/80, fasting blood sugar of **above** 100 mg/dl, or low HDL [**below** 50 mg/dl]).

Y N DK   My father has or had diabetes or metabolic syndrome (three of the following symptoms: high triglycerides [**above** 150 mg/dl], waist measurement of **more than** 40 inches, blood pressure of **at least** 135/80, fasting blood sugar of **above** 100 mg/dl, or low HDL [**below** 40 mg/dl].

Y N DK   One of my grandparents on my mother's side has or had diabetes or metabolic syndrome.

Y N DK   One of my grandparents on my father's side has or had diabetes or metabolic syndrome.

Y N DK   One or more of my siblings or half siblings has or had diabetes or metabolic syndrome.

Y N DK   One or more of my blood-related aunts or uncles has or had diabetes or metabolic syndrome.

My own risk factors:

Y N DK   My fasting blood sugar is or has been **too high,** above 100 mg/dl.

Y N DK   My bad blood LDL cholesterol is **above** 100 mg/dl.

Y N DK   My blood triglycerides have been **above** 150 mg/dl.

Y N DK   My good blood HDL cholesterol is **below** 45 mg/dl (for men) or 55 mg/dl (for women).

Y N DK   I am taking a blood sugar–lowering medication or using insulin.

Y N DK   I carry my excess weight predominantly around the waist as opposed to the hips.

Y N DK   I would describe my exercise level as inactive.

Y N DK   I am a woman who has had a baby weighing more than 9 pounds at birth.

Y N DK   I experience frequent thirst more than other people I know.

Y N DK   I had an **elevated** fasting blood glucose level greater than 126 mg/dl while pregnant or was diagnosed with gestational diabetes.

PHENOTYPE E

The genetic connection:

Y   N   DK   My mother has or had depression, manic depression, or seasonal affective disorder, or is or was an emotional eater (one who eats when sad, happy, lonely, upset, bored, stressed, etc.).

Y   N   DK   My father has or had depression, manic depression, or seasonal affective disorder, or is or was an emotional eater (one who eats when sad, happy, lonely, upset, bored, stressed, etc.).

Y   N   DK   One of my grandparents on my mother's side has or had depression, manic depression, or seasonal affective disorder, or is or was an emotional eater.

Y   N   DK   One of my grandparents on my father's side has or had depression, manic depression, or seasonal affective disorder, or is or was an emotional eater.

Y   N   DK   One or more of my siblings or half siblings has or had depression, manic depression, or seasonal affective disorder, or is or was an emotional eater.

Y   N   DK   One or more of my blood-related aunts or uncles has or had depression, manic depression, or seasonal affective disorder, or is or was an emotional eater.

My own risk factors:

Y   N   DK   I am taking an antidepressant medication.

Y   N   DK   I eat more when I'm sad, happy, lonely, upset, bored, or stressed.

Y   N   DK   I tend to overeat when I am alone or in big groups, such as at parties.

Y   N   DK   There are times when I feel my eating is hard to control.

Y   N   DK   I rarely or never eat food early in the day and have trouble controlling what I eat at night.

Y   N   DK   I eat to calm my feelings.

Y   N   DK   Especially when stressed, I overeat even though my intention is to stop before I reach this point.

Y   N   DK   Extra time or personal time is nonexistent for me.

Y   N   DK   I sometimes feel ashamed of my eating.

Y   N   DK   My emotional eating does not seem to be related to hunger.

PHENOTYPE H (WOMEN ONLY)

The genetic connection:

Y   N   DK   My mother experienced menopause before age 50 either naturally or through surgery.

Y   N   DK   My mother dealt with significant symptoms such as hot flashes, mood swings, or sleep problems during pre-menopause or menopause.

Y   N   DK   My mother gained more than 20 pounds above the normal weight gain during pregnancy.

Y   N   DK   My mother had symptoms I would describe as premen-strual syndrome, such as food cravings, mood swings, or irritability.

Y   N   DK   My mother's mother experienced menopause before age 50, gained excess weight with pregnancy, or had symp-toms I would describe as premenstrual syndrome.

Y   N   DK   Other female blood relatives experienced menopause before age 50, gained excess weight with pregnancy, or had symptoms I would describe as premenstrual syn-drome.

My own risk factors:

Y   N   DK   I have gained more than the recommended weight gain for pregnancy and kept it on.

Y   N   DK   I experience symptoms I would describe as premenstrual syndrome.

Y   N   DK   My eating increases or changes significantly with my menstrual cycle.

Y   N   DK   I experience food cravings during the two weeks before my period.

Y   N   DK   My weight seems to increase the older I get.

Y N DK   I had a pear-shaped body at one time but now have an apple-shaped body.

Y N DK   I am female and approaching age 50.

Y N DK   I am currently taking female hormones such as estrogen and/or progesterone or testosterone for symptoms such as hot flashes, mood swings, or sleep problems.

Y N DK   I am experiencing hot flashes, mood swings, and night sweats.

Y N DK   I have gained 10 pounds or more excess weight with menopause.

SCORING

Go back through the quiz and count the number of YES statements for each phenotype. Enter the number for each phenotype separately.

Phenotype A _____

Phenotype B _____

Phenotype C _____

Phenotype D _____

Phenotype E _____

Phenotype H _____

The category with the highest number of points is your phenotype.

My personal phenotype is _____.

WHAT IF THERE IS A TIE?

1. If your scores are tied between two or more phenotypes, total your scores for "The genetic connection" questions *only*. See if

(continued on next page)

there is a clear phenotype choice based on the family history answers alone. If there is, this phenotype is the diet plan you should follow.

2. If there is not a clear phenotype choice based on family history questions, total your scores for the "My own risk factors" questions. See if there is a clear phenotype choice based on your personal risk factors alone. If there is, this phenotype is the diet plan you should follow.

3. If a tie still exists, look at the diets, the food lists, and the menus, and choose the one you are most comfortable with. Either diet will work for weight loss and to reduce your health risks.

WEIGHT GAIN TRIGGERS: THE LINK BETWEEN YOUR ENVIRONMENT AND YOUR WEIGHT

Now that you have determined your phenotype, you will be eager to move to the chapter that matches it. Yet to do so without taking full stock of the factors that activate your fat-causing genes is premature. This is where "nurture"—an element over which you have almost complete control—comes in.

The environments where you live and work and the ways in which you interact with them propel you either toward or away from weight loss and health by activating or "triggering" genes. Food choices, stress or relaxation, portions, risky behaviors, exercise or the lack of it—all turn on or off your genes. Scientific literature calls these "environmental triggers" be-

WEIGHT GAIN TRIGGERS

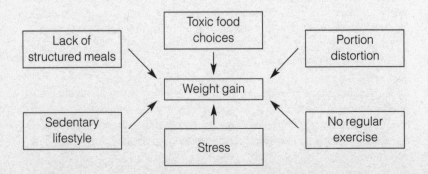

cause they begin outside you. Negative triggering puts a series of gene-based chemical events into motion that lead to weight gain and disease. Positive triggering does the opposite. If you couldn't switch from negative to positive, fat really would be your fate.

These six aspects of your present environment may be triggering your genes into derailing health and weight loss efforts. It's not as simple as "too many calories, too little exercise." Yes, these triggers precipitate a flood of chemicals that modify the way you metabolize food and determine whether you store or burn excess calories, but they also lead to weight gain in other ways. For example, the hormone cortisol, which stress increases, changes the receptors on fat cells in the abdominal region and promotes fat storage there. Whereas sitting still reduces the metabolic rate, burns fewer calories, and stores more fat, exercise speeds the metabolic rate, increasing fat burning capacity for twelve to twenty-four hours even after the exercise is finished and reduces fat storage. Portion distortion sets you up for ongoing weight gain by increasing the number and size of fat cells. Lack of structured meals and toxic food choices starve your body of antioxidant chemicals, provoking stress responses and inciting the inflammation associated with diabetes and heart disease. Unaided by minerals supplied by antioxidant-rich foods, blood pressure tends to rise.

Likely, several of these weight triggers are very familiar. Countless times you may have considered their role in your weight gain. Perhaps your response is: *But I can't change where I work. I don't have more time. I can't afford fresh fruits or vegetables.* Yes, some of these negative triggers are imposed on us. Certainly processed food, stress, sedentary deskwork and driving are practically unavoidable in our modern lives. Nonetheless, if you ignore the factors that are triggering your weight gain while dieting, you will not succeed in keeping it off. You have more power than you think you do. Positive triggers can counteract negative ones, and this book demonstrates how in subsequent chapters. But first you have to recognize your negative triggers and their role in your weight gain. You have to become accountable.

WEIGHT TRIGGER QUIZ

Taking the following Weight Trigger Quiz will help you focus on those negative influences that most pertain to you. Examining your routine honestly, and factoring in its effect on your body chemistry, will leave no doubt as to how your opportunities for weight loss are being sabotaged. Please read each statement under every category and answer "true" or "false" as it relates to you.

TOXIC FOOD CHOICES

T   F   I prefer fried foods and eat them regularly.

T   F   I love sweets and treats and eat them often.

T   F   I drink regular soft drinks and drink them often.

T   F   I eat at fast-food restaurants three or more times per week.

T   F   I eat chips, crackers, or cookies regularly.

T   F   I rarely prepare food at home.

T   F   I don't like vegetables or I rarely eat them.

T   F   I don't like many fruits or I rarely eat them.

T   F   My regular beverage choices contain calories such as those from juice, fruit drinks or sodas.

T   F   I drink more than three alcohol drinks per day (men) or more than two drinks per day (women).

LACK OF STRUCTURED MEALS

T   F   Meals prepared and eaten at home are rare.

T   F   I regularly skip at least one meal a day.

T   F   A majority of my calories come from snack foods.

T   F   I eat more food when alone.

T   F   I don't have time to prepare meals.

T   F   My work requires long hours.

T   F   I work a night shift.

T   F   I don't plan what I'm going to eat in advance.

T   F   I have been on many diets to lose weight.

T   F   I'm constantly going on and off a diet.

PORTION DISTORTION

T   F   As far as meals or snacks go, the bigger the better.

T   F   I like restaurants where it's all you can eat.

T   F   A meal is not complete without dessert.

T   F   I am a definite member of the clean-plate club.

T   F   When eating out, I usually go for the largest portions.

T   F   At fast food restaurants, I usually get a meal combo or super-size.

T   F   I don't like to share portions at restaurants.

T   F   In restaurants, I don't ask for doggie bags because I eat what's served.

T   F   I don't pay much attention to the serving size on food labels.

T   F   I sometimes worry that I won't get enough to eat.

STRESS

T   F   I would classify myself as a stress eater.

T   F   I often feel as if I have no personal time.

T   F   Eating is a way of relaxing for me.

T   F   I tend to eat the most calories toward the end of the day.

T   F   I eat more when I am frustrated, angry, sad, or lonely.

T   F   I rarely use exercise as a way to relieve stress.

T   F   There are never enough hours in the day to do what I need to do.

T   F   I have frequent headaches, backaches, or stomach problems.

T   F   There have been major changes in my life recently such as marriage, a divorce, the death of a family member, a move, a new job, or a new baby.

T   F   I have difficulty sleeping.

INCREASINGLY SEDENTARY LIFESTYLE

T   F   My job involves three or more hours of computer work a day.

T   F   I sit and watch two or more hours of television a day.

T   F   I like to play video or computer games in my free time.

T   F   I would describe my daily activities as mostly sedentary.

T   F   I have significantly increased my screen time over the last two to three years.

T   F   My favorite leisure activities require sitting.

T   F   On the weekends, I spend three or more hours a day sitting at the computer.

T   F   After dinner at night, I like to relax by watching television or working/playing on the computer.

T   F   I sit and watch an average of three or more movies a week.

T   F   I have gained weight since increasing my screen time.

NO REGULAR EXERCISE

T   F   I would describe my activity level as sedentary.

T   F   I do little or no purposeful exercise.

T   F   I don't enjoy exercise.

T   F   I have tried exercise programs but always quit.

T   F   I have an injury or disability that prevents me from exercising.

T   F   I don't have time for exercise.

T   F   I spend a majority of my day in the car or other vehicle.

T   F   Extra time or personal time is nonexistent for me.

T   F   Exercise is not a priority for me.

T   F   I have gained weight since stopping an exercise program.

SCORING

Go back through your quiz, and counting each true statement as 1 point, add up the total points for each category separately. Record below.

Toxic food choices   _____

Lack of structured meals   _____

Portion distortion   _____

Stress   _____

Increasingly sedentary lifestyle _____

No regular exercise   _____

The categories with the highest number of points are your most destructive triggers, the habits that most promote weight gain. Now that you know, you can make changes to counteract them.

Your phenotype diet + Positive triggers = Your prescription for weight loss

Write down your phenotype   _____

Check the positive triggers you most need to achieve

        _____ Best food choices

        _____ Structured meals

        _____ Portion Control

        _____ Less stress

        _____ Active lifestyle

        _____ Regular exercise

Each phenotype chapter explains how best to control weight triggers. Following the recommendations for food choices, structured meals, and portion control in the phenotype diets will counteract the three food-related negative triggers. Likewise, your phenotype chapter will explain how to offset non-food-related triggers with less stress, active lifestyle, and regular exercise.

Before turning to the chapter on your Phenotype to begin this exciting just-for-you weight loss program, please have a look at our easy tips on how to use this book in the following brief chapter.

CHAPTER 3

The Road Map to
Your Phenotype Diet

TIPS ON HOW TO USE THIS BOOK

You've found your phenotype and pinpointed the routine triggers that undermine both your weight and your health. Now it's time to tackle those triggers.

This "how-to-use" section is brief but essential, as it will help you make best use of your phenotype diet, as will the Appendices, Resources, and References. The description that follows explains why we designed the book as we did. It also demonstrates how eating and living differently can immediately increase your control over your genetic destiny. Each phenotype diet includes the following steps.

STEP ONE: UNDERSTANDING YOUR PHENOTYPE

This section explores what promotes weight gain in your particular phenotype. It characterizes the challenge that your phenotype-based diet is designed to overcome. Reading it will help you understand the scientific scope of the task ahead of you—"rewiring" your genetic responses to work for rather than against weight loss. It will also inspire you to avoid or manage your weight-related health risks, be they addiction, high blood pressure, cardiovascular disease, diabetes, emotional eating, or hormonal changes.

STEP TWO: KEEPING A FOOD RECORD

Many studies confirm that dieters who keep a written record of what they eat lose more weight. Those who keep a Food Record also tend to keep it off. This has also been our experience during twenty years of nutrition consulting. Food recording works because it creates a communication loop to reinforce accountability—or self-responsibility, if you will.

When weight problems become chronic, eating can become the source of shame or self-delusion or both. Learning to communicate honestly with yourself about food will disclose where eating and lifestyle habits connect to your family, friends, work, and well being. It will also reveal how they can be improved. As you learn to outsmart your genes, keeping track of your progress will help you cope with your weak areas, better deal with setbacks, and best of all, provide an invaluable measure of your successes.

STEP THREE: DEVELOPING POSITIVE NONFOOD WEIGHT LOSS TRIGGERS

You identified the ways in which your environment goads your genes into weight gain in Chapter 2. In your phenotype chapter, Step Three will give you positive triggers to replace those negative triggers. Making *deliberate changes* to your behavior—changes you seriously consider and consciously initiate—will increase your accountability and contribute to your well-being. By following the suggestions, each geared to your phenotype along with the prescribed diet, you'll achieve the weight loss and better health you have been seeking.

STEP FOUR: FOLLOWING YOUR PHENOTYPE DIET

We scientifically crafted your phenotype-specific diet to turn off problematic genes and turn on health-giving genes. It has all the strategies you need for ridding yourself of the three remaining negative weight triggers: toxic food choices, lack of structured meals, and portion distortion. Each chapter's Phenotype Diet is divided as follows:

Focus Foods

Each Phenotype Diet features Focus Foods that work best to recondition that phenotype. This section explains how the dietary chemicals they contain work at a cellular level to prevent the unwanted gene expression that results in weight gain and disease. To help you make these Focus Foods an integral part of your daily and overall diet, the section also provides criteria for Focus Food Frequency. The Focus Foods for your phenotype will make an enormous difference in how you feel and will positively affect your success with weight loss. We've included the various Focus Foods in your sample menus as well as noted them in **bold** on your food list.

FAST TRACK Two Weeks

Your mental outlook and view of yourself are important to weight loss. Without positive self-esteem, the best weight loss diet can fail. That is why we start the Phenotype Diets with the *FAST TRACK* Two Weeks. (Phenotype As are an exception. Their health risks do not benefit from the initial *FAST TRACK* Two Weeks.) You will see a drop in your weight these first two weeks, providing a critical psychological lift and the motivation that you need to make upcoming deliberate lifestyle changes and move forward. Success breeds success. Use this motivation to continue with your Phenotype Diet.

You will lose weight quickly for a number of reasons. First, for these two weeks, you omit the two fist-size portions of "Sweets, Treats, and Alcohol" that you are allowed on the Phenotype Diets. In addition, the *FAST TRACK* Two Weeks is specifically based on your Phenotype Diet. Why for only two weeks? Because healthy weight loss and healthy eating are *not* about long-term deprivation nor about lowering your metabolism by eating too few calories for a lengthy period of time.

What's more, should you reach a plateau where you cannot seem to lose any more weight, you can return to the *FAST TRACK* to jump-start your weight loss again. By going back to the *FAST TRACK* for a week or two and kicking up your exercise a notch, your body will move past this plateau.

Portion Control

Your diet will tell you the number of proteins, carbohydrates, and fats to have at each meal or snack. The ratios are important because they recali-

How did you score in the "Portions" area of the Weight Trigger Quiz? Increased portion size is one of the single greatest environmental changes contributing to weight gain in the United States. Even though it may cost slightly more, buying foods packaged in single portions reduces the chances of overeating.

brate your system to encourage weight loss. To adjust the portions, we've based them on hand sizes. It couldn't be simpler. There's no need to weigh or measure anything. Your hand becomes your measuring tool, since you use your palm, fist, ½ fist, and thumb(s) to determine your portions.

 PALM

 FIST

 THUMB

Food Lists

For each meal, all you have to do is select food choices from the Food List in your phenotype chapter. Focus Foods for your phenotype are in **bold** on the Food List. We categorize foods into protein, carbohydrate, and fat selections and include freebies, which can be eaten in any quantity.

Sweets, treats, and alcohol are in a separate category. Yes, sweets, treats, and alcohol! If these diets were torture, few people would stick to them. The Phenotype Diets allow two fists 🖐 🖐 each week of whichever sweet, treat, or alcohol that you desire. You may use both fists at once, such as on a dish of your mother's homemade chocolate pudding when you visit her. Or you might prefer a glass of wine two times a week. It's your choice. By allowing these treats (including alcohol), you're much less likely to feel deprived and break your diet.

To use the two fists as treats, you don't have to subtract anything from your Phenotype Diet. These fists of treats were already included in the calculations.

> To use the two fists 🖐 🖐 as treats, you don't have to subtract anything from your Phenotype Diet.

Sample Menus

We provide sample menus to use or to build other menus around. NO-TIME Menus are quick and easy, and you can use precut, preprepped ready-to-eat items from your grocery. Anyone can follow them. MORE-TIME Menus aren't much more complicated but require more preparation. Don't forget to look in Appendix C for tasty recipes from your NO-TIME and MORE-TIME Menus.

Supplements

In addition to the focus foods, multivitamin/mineral supplements are required during any significant calorie restriction to insure proper intake of nutrients needed to run body processes and prevent the onset of diseases specific to each phenotype. Some additional supplements have merit in various circumstances. Others haven't been shown to be effective or sufficient studies haven't been done to evaluate their usefulness.

Sometimes the "placebo effect" (you think you're improving because you're taking what you believe is a real treatment) causes a person to feel better whether or not the supplement itself has any value. Unless "double-blind" studies have been conducted on a given supplement, its real merit is still unproven. A double-blind study evaluates results from two participating groups simultaneously, some taking an active supplement and others taking a placebo. The participants don't know which they are taking. Our supplement recommendations are based on results from studies that have shown both a benefit *and* studies that have been controlled for the placebo effect.

Remember, supplements may interact negatively with medications that you may be using; the most common are listed here as well. Before you start any new supplement, speak with your health care provider and discuss how the addition of a new supplement may affect over-the-counter (OTC) or prescription medications you currently take. To prevent problems and boost the diets' effectiveness, we relay cautionary background about a few of them.

HOW TO DEAL WITH PLATEAUS

Dieters rarely shed pounds at the same rate throughout a diet. All plateau now and then, reaching periods where weight seems to stick rather than continue to fall away. Don't let plateaus discourage you nor make you feel as though you have failed. They are normal.

We suggest weighing yourself only once a week. Any more frequently and the daily fluctuations due to fluid weight will drive you crazy. If your weight has not budged for two weeks in a row, you can either re-jump-start the process with the *FAST TRACK* Two Weeks, step up and mix up your exercise routine for two weeks, or combine both techniques. When you do the same exercise routine over and over your body is not being challenged to reach for a higher level of fitness. Either increasing the time that you work out, or adding another type of exercise into the mix—for example, 10 minutes of weights to your 20 minutes of aerobics—takes your body to a higher workout level and moves you beyond that plateau.

HOW TO CHOOSE A DAILY MULTIVITAMIN/MINERAL SUPPLEMENT

Name brand and cost are not critical factors. Knockoffs of the widely known brands may provide the same value. However, supplements are not regulated as to safety or ingredient composition. The following steps will help you investigate any supplement's worth:

1. *Investigate the safety and purity.* To aid you in making an informed decision, you can look at the latest data from independent research on www.consumerlab.com or www.supplementwatch.com. These two Web sites post the impartial test results that assure whether supplements actually contain the ingredients stated on the label. Check to see if the supplement brand you are considering is recommended.

2. *Look for the USP (United States Pharmacopeia) seal* on the product itself. The seal has nothing to do with safety or benefits of the product. However, it is your assurance that the product was tested and found to contain the ingredients listed and that they will dissolve.

3. *Compare DV percentages on the labels; look for nutrition information called Supplement Facts.* In purchasing your multivitamin/mineral supplement, aim for around 100 percent of the Daily Value, or "DV," for most vitamins and minerals with these exceptions:

Vitamin C: The new DV is 90 mg, and some researchers suggest up to 250 mg per day. Look for the 90–250 mg range.

Vitamin A: The preferable form of Vitamin A is beta-carotene. Make sure your product doesn't contain more than 4,000 IU of retinol (listed on labels as Vitamin A palmitate or acetate). Excess vitamin A may increase the risk of hip fractures, liver abnormalities, and even birth defects if taken during pregnancy. Look closely at the label and make sure that at least 20 percent of the vitamin A is from beta-carotene.

Vitamin K: Find a supplement with at least 120 mcg (micrograms), the new daily requirement. Since leafy greens are also good sources, if you take any type of blood thinning

(continued on next page)

medication or supplement, be sure to discuss your intake of Vitamin K from food and supplements with your physician.

Iron: Look for one with iron for premenopausal women and without iron for postmenopausal women and men (or no more than 8 mg for men).

Calcium: Be aware that no vitamin/mineral supplement will ever have enough calcium in a single pill or it would be the size of a large gumball. Meet calcium requirements through food and add an additional supplement if needed 1,200–1500 mg. Viactiv Soft Calcium Chews are an easy way to get 500 mg at a time.

Vitamin B12: If you're over 50, look for at least 2.4 mcg up to 6 mcg (the DV) since your stomach acid may not pull the B12 from food as it should.

4. In addition to your daily multivitamin/mineral supplement, we recommend additional vitamin C and vitamin E, as follows:

Vitamin C: Antioxidant vitamins such as vitamin C have been studied extensively regarding various health benefits. There is a large body of literature supporting vitamin C for stress, immunity, cancer risk reduction, and increased requirements for smokers and women taking oral contraceptives. Your multi may contain only 90 mg, which is the new DV. However, some research suggests that up to 250 mg may be required for optimal blood vitamin C levels. We recommend a vitamin C supplement of 250 mg for all phenotypes.

Vitamin E: There is significant evidence supporting the use of vitamin E supplements for stress, immunity, cancer risk reduction, and by dieters due to the lower calorie and fat intakes in weight control plans. For these reasons, in addition to the Focus Food sources, we recommend a vitamin E supplement of 200 IU for women and 400 IU for men for all phenotypes.

Remember in the *FAST TRACK* Two Weeks we talked about your mental outlook and how your view of yourself is important to weight loss? Without positive self-esteem, the best weight loss diet can fail. When you experience a plateau or a lapse, it can affect your self-esteem and make you feel like you should toss in the towel and give up. By going back to the *FAST*

TRACK Two Weeks, you can restart your weight loss and feel encouraged and motivated once again to keep going.

Phenotype Maintenance

Having a maintenance diet is critical to prevent backtracking to old habits and weight gain. When you have reached your desired weight goal, you will

If you get off track with your diet for some reason, don't be discouraged or give up. Everyone gives in to temptation sometimes. Setbacks happen. If you can identify what triggered the setback and learn from it, so much the better. If weight gain is the result, you can go back to the *FAST TRACK* until you drop the extra pounds, but not for more than two weeks.

transition to either the Phenotype Maintenance Diet for Women or the Phenotype Maintenance Diet for Men, which are similar in design to your Phenotype Diet. This makes the transition easy, because your new habits will have become a way of life. As we mentioned before, the Phenotype Diet was right for you in the beginning and it's right now and for the future.

IN THE BACK OF THE BOOK

In the Appendices you'll find in-depth background on antioxidants, comparing fats, high-fiber foods, caffeine content in beverages, and mercury content in fish and seafood. A convenient list of no-prep foods will help you maintain your diet when you have no time at all. The "Ready Remedies" appendix tells you how to prime your diet by properly stocking your pantry, refrigerator, and freezer. The "Recipes" section provides you with detailed cooking instructions, the information you need about portions, and whether a dish requires NO-TIME or MORE-TIME preparation. The "Resources" section provides a list of companies and contact information for food items mentioned in the book, primarily in the sample menus.

LET'S GET STARTED

Together, these diets provide time-tested tools to help you build a new self. Remember, however, that this book is not a substitute for medical advice and care from your physician or other health care provider. Please don't hesitate to seek professional help. Now turn to the chapter that matches your phenotype to begin outsmarting your genes.

CHAPTER 4

The Phenotype A Diet

OUTSMARTING ADDICTION-
LINKED WEIGHT GAIN

Mary Ann's Story

"Binge eating is really what I'm all about."

Twenty-eight-year-old Mary Ann works as a design assistant for an advertising firm. She has gained 30 pounds since college. The first thing she said to us was, "When I was in college, I gained the famous 'freshman fifteen,' then in my junior year went on a diet to lose it. I had to get the weight off before my roommate's wedding. All I ate for weeks were hard-boiled eggs and apples. I drank coffee in the morning and diet soft drinks all day for the caffeine to keep me going.

"I lost the fifteen pounds, but after the wedding I gained it right back. It was just too hard to keep up that kind of discipline . . . plus I was miserable and hungry. So, I started to eat whatever I wanted again. That is when the pattern of my weight going up and down all started. I'm constantly dieting and then bingeing on foods I know I shouldn't eat. I'm addicted to eating."

Bruce's Story

"I need something to help me get control of this eating thing."

"I was an alcoholic by age 34. My family knew it, my friends knew it—it seems I was the only one who didn't know it. One night they all got together and began to tell me how my drinking was affecting them. I found out later that a meeting like that is called an intervention. It's a way to convince a person that they need help. Well, it sure got to me to see the people I love, crying and unhappy because of me. So, I went into treatment and I've been basically sober now for a year. The problem is I've gained nearly 40 pounds. I need something to help me get control of this eating thing."

Food had become Bruce's new addiction. Without realizing it, he was using dietary chemicals from food the same way he had used alcohol—to modify his brain chemistry.

If you are overweight and a Phenotype A, you answered "yes" to some of these statements in the Phenotype Assessment:

- I gained significant weight after stopping the use of drugs or alcohol.
- There are times when I feel that I cannot control what or how much I am eating.
- I often eat alone because I feel embarrassed about how much I am eating.
- After eating, I often feel depressed, disgusted, or guilty about overeating.
- I binge-eat on an average of two days a week.
- I have frequent cravings for salty, sweet, or fatty foods.

STEP ONE: UNDERSTANDING YOUR PHENOTYPE

Phenotype As gain weight in association with a genetic tendency for addiction. If you are a binge eater or if you have gained weight after treatment for alcohol or drug addiction, this is your phenotype. Addictive eating is a three-pronged problem consisting of your genes, your behaviors, and the chemical effects of the foods you overeat. Research has established a strong connection between weight gain and addiction. Interdependent, they both stem from common genetic groupings that we call Phenotype A.

There is one other group that can also benefit from the Phenotype A Diet—former tobacco users. Tobacco is an addictive substance and the nicotine in tobacco speeds up the metabolism. When you stop using it, you gain weight partly because the withdrawal of nicotine slows down your metabolism. In addition, food often becomes a good substitute for the hand-to-mouth movement involved in smoking, resulting in additional caloric intake and weight gain. Although former smokers may not have the same genetic connection as other Phenotype As, they do have the addiction and the cravings that contributed to their weight gain, and the Phenotype A Diet helps control these issues.

Your Brain Chemicals and Substance Abuse

As contrasted to nonaddictive people, who have "feel-good" genes that optimize their neurotransmitters (brain chemicals) to produce a feeling of pleasure or well being, addictive people don't. Their ability to feel good is literally depressed, due to chemical imbalances in the brain. The "feel-good" genes of Phenotype As don't work, leaving them genetically predisposed to alcohol and drug abuse or gambling as well as other addictive patterns, such as binge-eating disorder. Binge eaters fall into two categories or subgroups, which we will discuss in a moment, but first let's look at how genes and their actions contribute to the addictive eating pattern.

Genetically, Phenotype As may have low levels of the neurotransmitters dopamine or serotonin, or they may have too few receptors for these neurotransmitters on their brain cell surfaces. This leads to a craving for a substance or behavior that alleviates the "low" they are experiencing. In other words, a person whose genes leave him or her with less dopamine or serotonin, or with fewer brain receptors for dopamine or serotonin, will naturally strive to find a "high" some other way, all too often through substance abuse. Phenotype As are trying to achieve a level of pleasure that their genes and behaviors have put out of reach.

This pattern is evident throughout substance abuse research. For example, psychiatrist Nora Volkow and colleagues reported that compulsive overeaters have lower dopamine receptor availability, just like drug addicts. In her research, this dopamine deficiency contributed to their risk of developing compulsive or binge eating.

Dr. Kenneth Blum named the possible genetic or inherited condition associated with addiction the *Reward-Deficiency Syndrome.* Low brain dopamine levels, caused by a version of the dopamine D2 receptor gene, may produce a higher risk for addictive eating as well as obesity, alcoholism, substance abuse, and other behavioral addictions such as gambling, shopping, and even sex. In Reward-Deficiency Syndrome, a disruption of the brain chemical dopamine results in feeling anxious and/or angry, or in a craving for a substance or a behavior that alleviates the negative emotions. In this theory, genetic anomalies (variations) in the D2 gene can lead to a self-sustaining pattern of abnormal cravings.

If your parents or other close relatives have been addicted, you may have inherited the genes we've just described and the risk that goes with them. Overweight people with binge-eating disorder are significantly more likely to have a family history of substance abuse than the general population. Therefore, we may see a parent who is addicted to alcohol and a child, even an adult child, who is overweight and a binge eater.

Which Binge Eater Type Are You?

According to research in the *International Journal of Eating Disorders*, binge eaters divide into two subgroups—*chronic dieters* and *depressive eaters*—as we mentioned previously. In the first subgroup are chronic dieters, accounting for 63 percent. *Chronic dieters* such as Mary Ann try diet after diet, all very restrictive, but binge eating between diets prevents them from losing significant weight permanently. Mary Ann was eating nothing but apples and hard-cooked eggs to lose weight until this lack of structured meals and severe deprivation led to boredom and overeating. Many of our clients, including Mary Ann, have told us that breaking a restrictive diet often leads to a binge. Dieting restrictively actually is part of the problem, rather than the solution.

That is why the Phenotype A Diet contains two fists of sweets, treats, or alcohol each week, with some limitations. If you are a recovering alcoholic like Bruce, you obviously can't use your two fists on alcohol. If eating pizza actually causes you to lose control over your eating, it isn't a good idea to indulge in pizza until you feel more in control. So substitute other recommended foods, such as Focus Foods, for your addictive substances. Getting away from dieting restriction will lead away from the "I'm on a diet—I'm off a diet" mentality, which is critical to stopping binge eating.

Joanna's Story

"I was so down and depressed, but the depression sure didn't depress my appetite!"

"I have friends who stop eating when they're upset and depressed. But not me. When my husband and I started going to counseling, I couldn't stop eating even if I tried. Eating was definitely my comfort. Food was like a warm blanket on a cold, rainy night. After a painful and sometimes hurtful discussion with my husband, I often felt guilty and remorseful about the things I had said. Then I would binge eat and *feel temporarily better. When the therapist suggested that I was depressed, I couldn't believe it.*

When I took the Phenotype Assessment, I knew immediately that I was definitely a Phenotype A because my mother was an alcoholic. I never thought much about how her moods and behaviors had affected me until I was in a bad marriage like she had been and was eating instead of drinking. Just knowing that connection existed was helpful in changing my patterns. And the combination of the right diet, medication, and therapy was my salvation."

Joanna typifies the second group of binge eaters, the *depressive eaters,* who account for 37 percent of Phenotype As. Her psychological issue became a food issue. The "guilt/remorse" syndrome turned to "good food/bad food." And the alternating good food/bad food thinking added a need to deprive herself, what we call "restrictive" dieting. Depression like Joanna's is seen more in women than in men, runs in families, and tends to reoccur periodically. In this gene-based subgroup, mood, anxiety, or personality disorders produce greater eating and weight obsession, relationship problems, and continued weight gain. Stressful events can precipitate or aggravate an episode in someone who has a family history of depression. The cycle often includes a low-self-esteem component, like this:

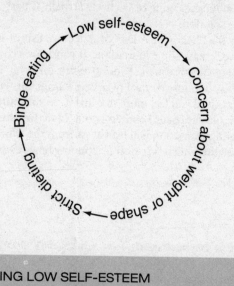

OVERCOMING LOW SELF-ESTEEM

- *Rethink your perception of your body size and shape.* Most women negatively focus on the weight issue without thinking about the rest of the story such as height differences. Mary Ann, for example, was always disappointed in herself when she looked at fashion models in magazines. Through discussions with her therapist, Mary Ann learned to accept her height and shape and not to compare herself to touched-up photos of people who are up to a foot taller than she with completely different and more than likely unrealistic body shapes. Sometimes people can accomplish feelings of acceptance on their own; other times they require the help of a therapist.

- *Accept and enhance inherited traits, such as height and bone size.* One thing that helped the process was Mary Ann's looking at pictures of her mother when she was Mary Ann's age, so that she could actually see her genetic inheritance. She made a decision to play up her best features and let go of the rest.

- *Make a list of your strengths.* Turn negative thoughts into positive ones. When you compare your weaknesses to someone else's strengths, you will always come up short. You can only really compare yourself against yourself, since you are unique and no one has your exact same genetic package.

- *Reinforce and augment your positive self-esteem by incorporating the impressions of good friends and family members who love you.* Joanna's best friend helped her focus on her beautiful traits, such as her thick, curly hair, her bright blue eyes, and her volunteer work with a Girl Scout troop, where she could help the girls learn how to develop positive food associations and behaviors.

There is no such thing as an ideal body size or shape, just a completely unique you. Celebrate your uniqueness. If you constantly compare your worst to someone else's best, you will always fall short. Positive self-esteem will help to break the cycle of dieting and binge eating.

For depressive Phenotype As, replacing nutrient-deficient foods that exacerbate depression with foods that are satiating and nutritious is critical for putting an end to binge eating. By focusing on *healthy eating* rather than another restrictive diet, Joanna, as an example, reduced her binge-eating episodes, and began to feel better about herself.

If depression runs in your family, or you have been feeling depressed, please analyze your depression risk:

HOW HIGH IS YOUR DEPRESSION RISK?
PLEASE ANSWER THE FOLLOWING QUESTIONS:

1. Are activities that you have always found pleasurable no longer enjoyable?
2. Do you feel tired all the time without any apparent reason?
3. Do you sleep more than usual or have insomnia?
4. Do you feel like eating all the time, especially sweets, or has your appetite decreased significantly?
5. Do tasks that used to seem simple now seem very difficult?
6. Are you avoiding friends and crowds?
7. Are you having a very hard time getting over a loss or trauma in your life?
8. Are you feeling hopeless and worthless, as though life is not worth living?
9. Are you unable to go to work or keep up with responsibilities that are part of your daily life because you feel bad and don't know why?

If you answered yes to four or more of these questions, and especially if you answered yes to Question 8, it's time to see your physician or a mental health professional. Depression is not a character flaw; it's a very treatable medical condition. Research has shown that talk therapy and medication work together to correct the neurotransmitter changes associated with depression, improve your mood, and help you deal with stressful life events. A therapist or counselor, psychologist, or psychiatrist can provide the right combination of talk therapy and medication that is most effective in dealing with depression or other mood disorders.

Please remember that if you are binge eating, you need to find a therapist who has experience with eating disorders. The longer binge eating continues, the harder it may be to change. A therapist can help you understand the feelings that lead to craving and bingeing so you don't have to stuff them down with food. Until you get to the root of what prompts your binge eating, any weight you lose is likely to return.

This link between depression and substance abuse is well established in both men and women. Though depressed men are more likely than women to meet the criteria for substance abuse, depressed women are significantly more likely than men to succumb to eating disorders. As many as half of all people with binge-eating disorder have been depressed in the past, according to the National Institute of Diabetes and Digestive and Kidney Disease, and many binge eaters say that being angry, sad, bored, or worried can cause them to binge eat.

Addictive eating is very different from emotional eating (Phenotype E), due primarily to the genetic connection to addiction. Also, whereas Phenotype Es eat to calm their feelings, Phenotype As crave and eat to block emotions. For example, a Phenotype E reaches for a candy bar to comfort herself after a fight with her boss. That one candy bar doesn't lead to a binge, however, but it could become a frequently repeated way to cope with emotions. A Phenotype A, on the other hand, feels bad and eats cookie dough ice cream to numb her feelings—first a bowlful, then the entire container. She eats to block or numb emotions, not to achieve a change in emotions. Again, we don't know whether depression causes the bingeing or bingeing causes the depression, but we do know that neurotransmitters are involved, helped along by poor eating habits and other behaviors.

Dopamine problems may not result only in depression. Sometimes neurotransmitter deficiencies manifest as other mood disorders. What is consistent among Phenotype A's, however, is the genetic history of mood disorders and addiction.

Chantel's Story

"There were times I'd wake up wired in the middle of the night and couldn't stop thinking about my latest worry."

"I always thought I was just a worrier. I'd feel keyed up and unable to relax. At times it would come and go, and at times it would be constant. It could go on for days. I'd worry about what I was going to fix for a dinner party or what would be a great present for somebody. I just couldn't let it go and move on to something else. When I would binge, I would worry about that and how I was going to stop and who would find out.

"I'd also have terrible trouble sleeping. There were times I'd wake up wired in the middle of the night and couldn't stop thinking about my latest worry. I also had trouble concentrating, even reading the newspaper or a novel. Sometimes I'd even feel a little light-headed. My heart would race or pound. And that would make me worry more. I was always imagining things were worse than they really were. When I got a stomachache, I'd think it was an ulcer or cancer. When my problems were at their worst, I'd miss work and feel just terrible about it. Then I worried that I'd lose my job. My life was miserable until I got treatment."

Chantel wasn't depressed, but she had all the symptoms of an anxiety disorder. Working with a therapist, taking antianxiety medications, and following the Phenotype A Diet have helped to decrease Chantel's binge-eating episodes significantly. She used to binge three to four times a week but since beginning treatment and the diet has reduced that to an average of once every few months. As she continues this treatment plan and diet, Chantel can reach the point where her need to binge dissipates entirely.

How Your Eating Became Addictive

Greg's Story

"When I stopped drinking, I started eating."

"I'm definitely an addict and probably have been since I was young. I started drinking alcohol about age thirteen. My parents weren't home in the afternoon. I was alone, unhappy, and I liked the way it made me feel . . . it was an escape. I only quit drinking three years ago." Greg just turned 43, and he has lost his wife and children, several jobs, and thirty years of life due to his addiction.

Now sober, Greg has a good job, but, like Bruce, wanted to stop his new compulsive behavior. *"Without drinking, I couldn't seem to get enough desserts and sweets, and before long I had gained fifty pounds. Staying away from alcohol is hard, and I've slipped a few times. But food is legal, it's always there, and everyone eats. So it's become my new addiction."*

Can food really become as big and destructive a substance abuse problem as alcohol and drugs? For food to be considered "addictive," it has to meet the same criteria as other addictive substances.

YOU ARE AN ADDICT IF . . .

- You feel as though you've lost control.
- The substances you abuse produce a change in mood such as sedation, relaxation, or euphoria.
- These mood effects reinforce the substance use; that is, the feelings aroused by the substance make you want to use it again.
- You think about the substance all the time.
- You use the substance compulsively.

- You feel as though you *must* have the substance.
- Substance use continues despite negative consequences.
- You use substances on a regular basis and at specific times during the day.
- When you don't have the substance or can't get it, the desire to have it increases.

As you can see, compulsive eating is very similar to other substance addictions. However, food, in addition to leading to compulsive food-seeking and food-using behavior, must meet one more criterion to be like drugs or alcohol: *it must also affect brain chemicals.* Though to a lesser degree, food does alter brain chemicals. In a series of chemical reactions, dietary chemicals create precursors, substances that form other substances. These get into the brain, thus affecting the overall brain chemical balance. For example, amino acids from proteins or carbohydrates are precursors of the brain chemicals dopamine and serotonin. And caffeine, a central nervous system stimulant, affects dopamine levels in the brain to produce that temporary state of alertness, concentration, and energy.

Craved foods and trigger foods are often different. A craving is a desire for a certain food. Phenotype As crave foods that will affect, however temporarily, their brain chemistry. Trigger foods are different in that they precede or trigger eating out of control. A binge usually follows.

Here we must distinguish between cravings and trigger foods. Cravings don't necessarily precipitate a binge. Trigger foods do, and cravings sometimes turn into triggers, especially if that food has been restricted. For some of our clients, the trigger food is French fries, for others it's ice cream, and for others brownies or cookies. (Usually trigger foods are specific, such as chocolate, rather than general, such as all sweets.)

Whether craving or trigger, both issue from combined genetic vulnerability and "environmental" or exterior cues. The craving for certain foods, like the craving for drugs and alcohol, seems to spring not just from the physiological need for a dopamine stimulus on the inside but also from exposure and associations on the outside. As a Phenotype A, you are already functioning on a "feel-good" deficit, as explained, which makes you yearn to feel better. You may associate a substance that made you feel better in a past situation with making you feel better again. So, for example, going to the same bar where you used to drink with your friends may make you desire alcohol. Or a drive by a doughnut store may fill you with an irresistible urge to eat doughnuts. The initial longing turns into a craving, a craving you may indulge. Satisfying the craving with a couple of chocolates isn't a problem unless it precipitates or "triggers" out-of-control eating, i.e., a binge. That is addiction.

Identifying Your Addiction

Teresa's Story

"I knew that I was addicted to sugar."

"I just couldn't seem to control the amounts I ate once I got started. I would avoid it entirely for weeks, and then if someone brought doughnuts to the office, I might eat one in the morning. But then they would just call my name the rest of the day, and sometimes I'd even stop and buy a dozen Krispy Kremes on the way home and eat them all that night. When I went on the Phenotype A Diet and kept my binge-eating Food Record, I learned I could eat some foods containing sugar but not others. I did better if it was combined with some protein and fat . . . that seemed to take the edge off. I also learned how frequently and what types of sugary foods I could eat without bingeing, which made me feel a lot more in control."

Many people claim, like Teresa, to be addicted to sugar. Is that addiction or availability? The average American consumes 300 to 400 calories of added sugar each day, more than our prehistoric ancestors ate in their short lifetime. It adds up to more than 100 pounds a year. Sugar and other sweeteners are definitely more available today and relatively cheap. Note how often corn syrup is the number one ingredient in sweet foods. But is sugar really addictive? Some researchers argue yes, others no. To the extent that taste affects cravings, genetics plays a role.

Researcher Dr. Adam Drewnowski from the University of Washington suggests that taste preferences and taste rejections may be inherited. His research categorizes people as nontasters, medium tasters, and supertasters based on the number of the tongue's taste buds and the reaction to the bitter taste of 6-*n*-propylthiouracil, also called PROP. With more taste buds, supertasters receive a more amplified impression of taste; they "turn up the volume" of bitterness in grapefruit juice, broccoli, cabbage, coffee, and some soy products. Nontasters are less discriminating due to fewer taste buds and may actually need more food and more sugary, fatty foods to get a satisfaction response. They are the group at greatest risk for obesity.

Our client Don is a good example. He is a quantity-over-quality kind of guy, a nontaster who puts hot sauce on nearly everything. He says, "The hotter the better" and calls most foods "too bland." No matter what foods Don eats, he always overeats. He tried one diet after another with no lasting success until he tried the Phenotype A Diet.

Whether supertaster, nontaster, or somewhere in between, the truth is that your body doesn't distinguish between natural sugar and added sugar in foods. In other words, it's not the sugar itself that produces the binge; it's the connection of sugar to desirable things. Many researchers believe that "addictive" foods such as sugar carry emotional associations that make them special or rewarding or even temptingly illicit.

In addition to the challenge of addiction itself is the fact that foods Phenotype As such as Teresa and Don typically crave are high-calorie, low-nutrient foods, and overeating them can lead to weight-related diseases. When you really examine frequent cravings, you'll notice they aren't always for sugar. Sweets such as chocolate, ice cream, cookies, and cake are among the so-called forbidden foods, but pizza, chips, and French fries are not sweet. Notice, however, that these cravings do have one ingredient in common: fat! As Dr. Drenowski and others have demonstrated, many food addicts claim that they have a sweet tooth, but if they truly craved simply sugar, they would want lollipops, Life Savers, or cotton candy, since they are almost 100 percent sugar.

This, however, is rarely the case, except in young children. Around puberty, young women seek out sugar/fat combos, driven by estrogen to store fat and prepare for possible pregnancy. These preferences may persist into adulthood. Most so-called sugar cravers hunger for chocolate candy, pies, cakes, or cookies, which are composed mainly of fat with sugar added. Young men begin to prefer the combination of protein and fat. This is spurred by the need to build muscle, and this inclination persists into adulthood. Protein foods such as nuts, cheese, fatty meats, and pizza are really higher in fat than protein (approximately 50 to 60 percent of their calories come from fat). Even what people call "salt cravings" are often fat cravings. The number one salty food craving is for potato chips, in which approximately 60 percent of calories come from fat.

Fat may seem like a reasonable food choice for Phenotype As, even if they are not aware of the reason, because high-fat foods deliver their own feel-good response by releasing endorphins, the same mood-enhancing neurochemicals released during exercise. Endorphins are morphinelike chemicals that exert analgesic effects by binding to opiate receptors on brain cells and increasing the pain threshold. They produce a powerful pleasure sensation. For both genders, high-fat food combinations can temporarily improve mood, but, eaten in excess amounts, as they often are by addictive types, they layer on the weight.

Degrees of Control over Eating

Addictive eating is different from drug and alcohol addiction because you can't abstain from food totally as you can from drugs and alcohol. Whether you think you are a sugar/fat addict, a carbohydrate/fat addict or a protein/

fat addict, what matters is not so much what the food is as the degree to which you are *in control of your eating.*

The goal is to satisfy the craving without triggering a binge. We know from experience that denying a craving doesn't work, even when people try to substitute healthier foods for craved foods. For example, many people and many diets maintain that sweet tooths like Teresa should simply eliminate foods that contain white flour or sugar. The problem, as we've said, is that severe food restriction can lead to a binge in Phenotype As, and the depressive, deprivation–indulgence cycle will recommence. If you crave chocolate and instead eat an apple, two bowls of cereal, and six graham crackers and *then* eat the chocolate, what have you accomplished? This is referred to as "eating around a craving."

DON'T COCK THE TRIGGER

If you overeat in response to a trigger food, it is important to substitute other foods from the Phenotype A Diet for that trigger food until you feel more in control. For instance, if you're a self-diagnosed sugar addict like Teresa, try adding some foods containing sugar that don't trigger binges, like fruit or fruit juice. Sugar-containing foods that are less likely to trigger overeating or bingeing are fruit, dried fruit, juice, yogurt, flavored milk, hot chocolate, BBQ sauce, jam or jelly, and even salad dressings.

If the craving for a certain food is infrequent and eating some of that food is satisfying without leading to a binge, it's okay to eat the craved food. *Eat only enough to satisfy the craving. This works only if the food is not a binge food. Getting to this point is a treatment goal.* Start with a small portion or a preportioned size. Then reevaluate the craving every few minutes by walking away, drinking a glass of water, and asking yourself if you're really hungry or are eating compulsively. The idea is to interrupt yourself and stop eating when you've had enough so that the potential for a binge is reduced—to become a *normal* eater.

How does normal eating differ from addictive eating? Nutritionist Francis Berg defines the difference between normal eating and addictive eating this way: Normal eating is *regular* eating. It means eating several times throughout the day and is governed by internal signals of hunger and satiety (feeling of fullness). In other words, normal eaters eat when they're hungry and stop when they're full or satisfied. Normal eating promotes clear thinking and mood stability. After eating, normal eaters feel good.

Thoughts of food, hunger, or weight occupy only a small part of their day, perhaps up to 15 to 20 percent, which includes considering what food to eat as well as when and how they are going to fix it.

Unlike normal eating, addictive eating, or what Berg calls a *dysfunctional pattern,* is very chaotic or sporadic. Bingeing, dieting, and regularly skipping meals characterize addictive eating. Addictive eaters consume significantly more than their internal signals of hunger or satiety would dictate. After eating, addictive eaters feel worse; they feel guilty about the amounts they have eaten, tired, moody, less able to concentrate, and increasingly preoccupied with food. Thoughts of food, hunger, and weight occupy 20 to 65 percent of their waking hours or more.

> Normal eaters think about food only up to 15 to 20 percent of the day, while binge eaters think about food 20 to 65 percent of the day.

So, as we compare the definition of normal eating with that of addictive eating, we see a clear progression in the intensity of compulsive food behavior and preoccupation with food and weight, similar to the compulsive changes we see in drug or alcohol addiction from first use to abuse and finally to dependence or addiction.

When does the addictive eater move from a "compulsion" to "addiction," actually starting to *binge-eat?* Some binge-eat every now and again, while those who meet the criteria for binge eating do so more regularly—at least two days a week for at least six months. How do you define a binge? A binge includes eating an amount of food within a two-hour period that is definitely larger than most people would eat, plus feeling a *lack of control over eating* during the binge. What does that mean in terms of real food? A binge might be eating half of a large bag of pretzels, a whole pint of ice cream, six cookies, and two candy bars.

> Binge-eating episodes are associated with at least three of the following:
>
> - Eating much more rapidly than normal
> - Eating until uncomfortably full
> - Eating large amounts of food when not physically hungry
> - Eating alone because of embarrassment by how much one is eating
> - Feeling disgusted with oneself, depressed, or very guilty about overeating

If you meet these criteria, *establishing a healthier pattern of eating is more important than dieting to lose weight.* Your first priority is to regain control of your eating and reduce the number and frequency of binge episodes. The Phenotype A Diet is designed to help you establish healthier eating patterns, but you may also need some help from a therapist who is experienced in treating binge-eating disorder.

Or, you may not yet be at the binge-eating phase. Perhaps following treatment for alcohol or drug addiction, you may have gained weight due to compulsive eating. The Phenotype A Diet will prevent food from becoming your addiction without triggering the overeating that follows more restrictive diets.

To recap, Phenotype As have genes that prime them for addiction and overeating or bingeing—either by leading to deficient neurotransmitters or deficient cell-surface receptors for neurotransmitters. Circumstances outside the body—food, exposures, and behaviors—can either boost the risk of addiction, or more optimally, they can repress it. Outsmarting those genes is the objective of the Phenotype A plan.

STEP TWO: KEEPING A FOOD RECORD

Getting control of addictive eating is a four-phase process. You need to:

- Analyze what kind of foods you crave.
- Determine what prompts your bingeing or overeating.
- Replace your nonfood weight gain triggers with weight loss triggers.
- Eat to restore the balance of neurochemicals (your brain chemicals) through food.

Note that the first two phases require data gathering and analysis. Therefore, keeping track of your addictive eating in a Food Record is an essential part of the plan. It will help you determine your cravings and what triggers your binge eating, as well as the frequency of your binges. Don, for example, who inherited the nontaster genes, had been overeating out of dissatisfaction. By charting his eating and analyzing his triggers, Don was able to stick with the foods on the diet. He lost 30 pounds and has kept it off for two years. Because the hot sauce he was so fond of was a *Freebie,* Don could stay on the diet long enough to change behaviors and realize success. And he could watch his level of satisfaction change as he kept his Food Record. Don't think you can skip this step.

Your Food Record can be as simple as this one.

ADDICTIVE EATING FOOD RECORD

DATE/TIME	WHAT YOU ATE	TRIGGER/CIRCUMSTANCE
9/2, 3:00 P.M.	Bag of M&M's	Boss was unhappy about a project so worked through lunch; worried about daughter starting school today; craved chocolate.
9/2, 9:00 P.M.	Entire bag of microwave popcorn	First time I stopped all day.
9/2, 9:30 P.M.	King-size Butterfinger bar	Just wasn't satisfied.

Be sure to write down what is going on at the time the eating, binge, or craving occurs. Later you can review to see if the cravings or overeating are related to weight triggers such as stress, too much time between eating, feelings of deprivation, or depression. Check to see if most cravings are sugar- and starch-based (carbohydrate), protein-based, or salt-based. In Teresa's case, as an example, the doughnut cravings were carbohydrate-based and were stress- and hunger-related. By keeping a Food Record, she learned to recognize her vulnerabilities and think constructively about helping herself.

STEP THREE: DEVELOPING POSITIVE NONFOOD WEIGHT LOSS TRIGGERS

Remember that when it comes to weight, your genetics and family history set you up for addiction and weight gain, but they by no means doom you. Ultimately, your routines—both food-related and non-food-related—can either move you toward addictive eating or toward a healthy lifestyle and diet. The Phenotype A Diet detailed later in this chapter changes the three food-related negative triggers from the quiz into positive triggers: best food choices, structured meals, and controlled portions. You can use your sweets and treats allowance to feel less deprived and more in control. The primary goal—to stabilize eating and reduce, then eliminate binge episodes—is helped along by the positive non-food-related weight loss triggers described in this section. You'll find that nurturing yourself in new ways will temper those neurotransmitter imbalance–driven desires.

Greg and Bruce scored very high on the Weight Trigger Quiz's nonfood categories—especially "Stress" and "No Regular Exercise." Mary Ann and Joanna both answered true to eight out of ten questions in the "Stress" category. They didn't get regular exercise, either. These indicators suggested lots of opportunity to develop better routines.

Sometimes weight gain triggers are situational, such as an argument with a spouse or a problem at work. Find healthful ways for diffusing tensions and releasing them in advance. Thus, when a situation seems as if it

PREEMPT YOUR EATING RESPONSE WITH THE FOUR Ds

Once you recognize the situations that are leading you to eat, as Don and Teresa did, you can change your reaction. To preempt the immediate eating that is literally a "gut reaction" to stress, hunger, feelings of deprivation, or depression, our clients and patients have relied on the **Four Ds,** used successfully in antiaddiction programs

- **Deep breathing:** Take ten slow, deep breaths in succession: breathe in to a count of ten, hold for a count of ten, and breathe out slowly to a count of ten.
- **Delay:** Wait at least ten minutes before eating; then see if you still feel like eating.
- **Drink water, coffee, or tea:** Have a glass of water or drink something hot, such as tea or coffee. Drinking helps satisfy the desire to eat.
- **Distraction:** Tailor your distractions to the source of the emotion. If it's stress that habitually makes you eat, schedule a "worry time" as Chantel did, or do a mechanical task such as pulling weeds or trimming shrubs to help clear your mind. If it's boredom, commit to a new and stimulating objective. If it's loneliness, call a friend or volunteer at a shelter or library. If you're angry, get physical and go for a brisk walk or clean a closet. Make a list of enjoyable or mechanical distractions you can do instead of eating, such as listening to music, gardening, doing laundry, playing your guitar or piano, cooking a meal for a sick friend, playing with a pet, or sending or answering e-mail. If you select your so-called distractions with attention, they can become passions—passions that will keep you from thinking about food.

may cause bingeing, you can consciously manage it differently. After a few times, that skill, rather than the binge behavior, can become a habit. Mental health therapists can be very helpful in identifying these patterns and finding ways to substitute more productive responses to reduce binge eating.

In other cases, weight gain triggers can be the result of abuse or neglect during childhood. That is why working with a therapist who understands and treats eating disorders is often both extremely important and beneficial.

When moving from negative to positive triggers in these categories, make deliberate changes, not perfection, your goal. We recommend making one change at a time and letting it become a habit before you start the next change. It typically takes three to four weeks for a change to become part of your life. Set nonfood incentives and reward yourself as you progress. Have a look at the following strategies for turning off your other nonfood triggers.

Reduce Your Stress

Examine your addictive eating behaviors in your Food Record. For example, Teresa realized that her bingeing was mostly about low self-esteem. Even though Greg stopped drinking alcohol to relax during stressful times, he saw that he had replaced it with candy and ice cream. This pattern of using or abusing a substance to deal with stress is difficult to break. The best strategy is to substitute other brain chemistry–changing activities such as exercise or relaxation techniques for food. Greg decided to do other activities, such as playing solitaire on his computer and doing crossword puzzles to help him deal with stress. Teresa, too, needed to make changes. She decided to add a walk after dinner and a bubble bath at 9 P.M. Find stress relievers like these that work for you and build them into your day. They will help break the stress–eating connection. Check out some of these other positive strategies for stress relief:

- Work with a therapist to determine the basis for your addictive eating and learn other positive strategies to deal with stress.
- Every time you feel stress getting the better of you, implement the Four Ds (see page 48). Remember Bruce, who went into treatment for his alcohol abuse and has now been sober for three years? He uses the Four Ds to help himself make a more conscious choice when he has a food craving. He tells us he knows the technique is working when he can resist his trigger food: nacho chips.
- Create a list of enjoyable distractions, other than food, and use them. Chantel began to schedule a biweekly nail appointment to

reward herself when she made it through that time frame without bingeing.

- Set aside a regular worry time. When stress tempts you to overeat or keeps you awake, put the thoughts aside until your scheduled worry time. Do not worry and eat at the same time.
- Schedule meals, separated from worry time. Make eating a conscious and deliberate event, not something you do when you're stressed. Keeping a meal schedule and eating regularly creates a feeling of energy rather than exhaustion. Whether it's a daily calendar, PDA, or computer that helps you plan and organize your meals, structure is something all of our clients say helps them maintain their diet.
- If you have a binge episode, remember that it is important to adjust your attitude from "I blew the diet" to "One mistake does not mean I'm a failure." What you are telling yourself is that for the rest of that day and tomorrow, you can make better choices.
- Keep only small-portion foods around the house, so you won't be tempted to overeat in response to stress. Supersized portions are a major recent change contributing to weight gain in the United States, and Phenotype As are particularly vulnerable because they have a history of binge eating. Keeping large portions of food available makes it more likely that you will overeat. Even though it may cost slightly more, buy foods packaged in single portions to reduce the chances of binge eating. Restaurants with buffets are not a good choice for Phenotype As since the many choices and large amounts of food are difficult to say no to. Greg told us that using his hand to gauge portions helped him feel in control when he ended up eating at a buffet.

Develop an Active Lifestyle

Joanna found that depression was a factor that triggered her binge eating and also triggered inactivity. By taking the depression risk quiz (page 38) and identifying the problem, she was able to understand and take control of her eating. In addition, she made a deliberate change toward getting more activity, which also improved her mood. Instead of calling for the daily report at work, she began to walk across the building and up the stairs to get it. She also found new ways at home to add activity, such as Roller-Blading around the neighborhood and going on her bike to yard sales every Saturday.

- Turn off the television or computer at least three nights a week and plan other more physical activities.

- Walk as much as you can—even if it's upstairs to eat lunch or down the hall to the water cooler. Set an alarm on your computer or PDA to remind you to get up and move.
- Schedule mini-outings during your day to increase your activity. Chantel made a deliberate change in her workday, taking a break and walking to a restaurant nearby for an iced tea before she went home. She added some activity and one of her Focus Foods (caffeine) during the critical afternoon time, when binge eating often starts.

Exercise Regularly

Exercise deflates stress, prevents boredom, and revs up metabolism for hours after the activity. It also produces endorphins, brain chemicals that help to improve mood. For addictive eaters, a daily workout will put brain chemicals on a more even keel.

- When you have the urge to eat, use exercise instead as a way to deal with stress or emotions. Greg joined a softball league and coached other sports during the off-season. Bruce started playing handball or racketball with his neighbor at the park near their houses.
- Keep trying activities until you find an exercise you enjoy or will do routinely. Mary Ann swore she had tried every exercise but never stuck with them. However, when they offered a yoga class at her office during lunch, she looked forward to the days it was held. She even asked the teacher if she could sign up for her class on Saturdays so she wouldn't miss an opportunity.
- Add frequent short bouts of exercise, such as ten minutes at a time. Ten minutes several times a day add up and break the routine of reaching for food. Most people can walk away from their desk and go somewhere, anywhere, to add activity during a long workday. Put on your pedometer (see below), walk around your building or block, and watch the steps add up.
- Buy a pedometer (good sources are www.digiwalker.com and www.accusplit.com) and wear it daily so you can see how far you currently walk. Set a goal to increase your distance by at least 100 steps each day. You'll be surprised how motivating it is. Some pedometers even show how many calories you are burning!

For many of you, these changes can easily be made on your own. But we know that for some of you these may seem like dramatic or even impossible changes. Because of their importance in changing your gene-based risks, please don't hesitate to seek help from a professional such as a registered dietitian, licensed mental health professional, physician, or certified personal trainer.

STEP FOUR: FOLLOWING THE PHENOTYPE A DIET

The Phenotype A Diet is built to help you succeed, treating both binge-eating disorder and weight gain after treatment for an alcohol/drug problem. It addresses the roots of the addictive eating problem by changing your eating cues, controlling your cravings, and helping you balance your brain chemicals so you feel more satisfied after eating.

First, we establish healthy eating patterns and avoid severe diet restrictions. These strategies decrease the number of binge-eating episodes and get you moving in a positive direction. This will enhance your self-image regardless of your weight. You won't feel like you're on a diet; you'll feel as though you've started a new and permanent healthy eating plan.

As you begin to recognize from your Food Record what your cravings and trigger foods are, you will understand the enormous benefit of eating foods that improve brain chemistry. The Phenotype A Diet works to readjust your brain chemicals—dopamine and serotonin—as much as possible through food. This means a regimen of approximately 50 percent carbohydrate, 20 percent protein, and 30 percent fat. If the carbohydrate level is too low, it'll trigger cravings. If you cut your protein intake lower, you won't get that slight boost in dopamine levels and you'll lose the satiety (feeling of fullness) that protein provides, which will cause you to overeat. If you don't eat enough fat, your mood will deteriorate and you'll also trig-

The Phenotype A Diet will change your diet to lose weight and control your addictive tendencies with the following critical changes:

- Adjustment of the distribution of calories to prevent hunger that may cause a binge.
- Adjustment of your protein/carbohydrate/fat ratio to balance your food–mood reactions.
- Use of caffeine to stimulate dopamine and maintain alertness.
- Identification and control of your cravings.
- Addition of planned snacks after Meal 2 and Meal 3, since bingeing most often occurs in the afternoon or evening.
- Addition of seafood and folic acid for mood stability.

ger overeating. And if you cut calories too severely to lose weight, the feeling of deprivation associated with strict dieting will trigger overeating once again. By contrast, this plan will change the person you are on a cellular level and assure you a much healthier future.

Focus Foods

The Phenotype A Diet has certain foods that are critical to the plan's design and success. They're called Focus Foods because research has shown them to be specifically beneficial to addictive eaters. As they can help make a difference in how you feel and positively affect your success, these Focus Foods are integral to your daily and overall eating plan. We've included them in your sample menus. Please make sure to add these foods into your diet on a regular basis (see Focus Food Frequency on page 54).

Caffeine: Caffeine boosts the body's production of dopamine and is a substance or food that in moderation is not harmful. A central nervous system stimulant, caffeine temporarily increases the brain's production of dopamine, not to the same degree as drugs or alcohol but enough to provide a temporary stimulation. There have now been dozens of well-controlled studies that have looked at caffeine and its effects. Many former addicts also find that caffeine helps them temporarily improve their focus and be more productive. We have included up to four servings of caffeine containing beverages in the Phenotype A Diet. If you have a nervous, shaky reaction to this much caffeine, start with a smaller dose and maintain it when you get to a comfortable level.

Protein: Protein is another food substance that temporarily raises brain levels of dopamine. By including protein, you add what is called satiety value to each meal and snack. Satiety is that feeling of satisfaction that you get after eating. Addictive eaters often overeat or binge mainly on carbohydrate foods and lack that feeling of satisfaction. Instead, they feel guilty after eating. We want to stop the guilt and give a feeling of control when you consume food. So you will see protein included in every meal or snack on the Phenotype A Diet.

Seafood, flaxseed meal, and walnuts: Oily fish such as salmon, mackerel, or tuna, walnuts, and flaxseed meal contain omega-3 fatty acids, which have a beneficial effect on mood and mood disorders. Research studies in *The American Journal of Psychiatry* and *Psychopharmacology Update* have concluded that people who eat fish are less likely to become depressed, due to their intake of omega-3 fatty acids. A country-by-country correlation between fish consumption and the rate of major depression found that in those countries where fish consumption was the highest, the rates of depression were lowest.

The mood benefits come almost entirely from the omega-3 fatty acids eicosapentaenoic acid (EPA) and docosahexaenoic acid (DHA). If you have never eaten much fish or seafood, now is a good time to try. Tuna comes in easy-to-use pouches that can be mixed with some chopped apple and a little light mayonnaise to make a great minimeal. If you are a vegetarian or don't like seafood, you can still get some benefits by using canola oil, soybean oil, soybeans, wheat germ, flaxseed meal, and walnuts. These foods contain the most abundant omega-3 fatty acid, alpha-linolenic acid (ALA). The human body converts up to 15 percent of ALA into DHA and EPA.

Folate foods: In people who are depressed, research has identified low blood levels of folate, one of the B vitamins, as a risk factor. Researchers at Harvard reported that low red blood cell folate levels have been found in 15 to 38 percent of adults diagnosed with depressive disorders. When their blood folate level was returned to the normal range by their eating foods containing folate or taking a supplement, symptoms of depression disappeared. Your blood folate level is associated with depression because folate is necessary in the last step in the conversion of tryptophan to serotonin in the brain. Low blood folate levels in depressed people have also been linked to a poor antidepressant response to the selective serotonin reuptake inhibitor (SSRI) drugs, such as Prozac and Zoloft. The best sources of folate

FOCUS FOOD FREQUENCY

FOOD ITEM	FREQUENCY
Caffeine-containing beverages	4 times daily, up to 600 mg
Protein foods	Each meal and snack
Seafood	3 times per week
Walnuts	3 times per week
Wheat germ	1 tablespoon 3 times per week
Canola or soybean oil	Daily when oil is needed
Flaxseed meal	1 tablespoon 3 times week
Folate foods	Daily

in food are green leafy vegetables, fruits, and other vegetables, and fortified cereals. As you'll see in the supplement discussion, a good multivitamin also includes the recommended level of folate listed as folic acid.

THE PHENOTYPE A DIET FOR WOMEN

Select your foods for each meal and snack from the Food List on page 57. Sample Menus using foods that fit the diet are on page 60.

Meal 1
1 Protein (any fist, ½ fist, or thumb[s] selection)
2 Carbohydrates
1 Fat
Freebie beverages

Meal 2
2 Proteins (1 palm **or** any 2: fist, ½ fist, or thumb[s] selections)
2 Carbohydrates
Freebie vegetables
1 Fat
Freebie beverages

Snack 1
1 Protein (1 palm **or** any fist, ½ fist, or thumb[s] selection)
1 Carbohydrate
1 Fat
Freebie beverages

Meal 3
2 Proteins (any 2: fist, ½ fist, or thumb[s] selections)
3 Carbohydrates
Freebie vegetables
2 Fats
Freebie beverages

Snack 2
1 Protein (any fist, ½ fist, or thumb[s] selection)
1 Carbohydrate
1 Fat
Freebie beverages

THE PHENOTYPE A DIET FOR MEN

Select your foods for each meal and snack from the Food List on page 57. Sample Menus using foods that fit the diet are on page 63.

Meal 1
1 Protein (any fist, ½ fist, or thumb[s] selection)
2 Carbohydrates
1 Fat
Freebie beverages

Meal 2
2 Proteins (1 palm **or** any 2: fist, ½ fist, or thumb[s] selections)
4 Carbohydrates
Freebie vegetables
1 Fat
Freebie beverages

Snack 1
1 Protein (any fist, ½ fist, or thumb[s] selection)
2 Carbohydrates
1 Fat
Freebie beverages

Meal 3
2 Proteins (any 2: fist, ½ fist, or thumb[s] selections)
5 Carbohydrates
Freebie vegetables
2 Fats
Freebie beverages

Snack 2
1 Protein (any fist, ½ fist, or thumb[s] selection)
1 Carbohydrate
Freebie beverages

FOOD LIST

Focus Foods are in **bold type.**

How much of each food should you eat? Use your hand as your guide. Eat the amount that you see; that is, the size of your fist, your palm, or your thumb.

 PALM

 FIST

 THUMB

Protein Sources

 Seafood. Poultry without skin, or lean cuts of meat such as loin, round, or cutlets of beef, pork, ham, veal, venison, lamb, etc.; cook by steaming, sautéing, broiling, or grilling. Meat alternative (tofu, tempeh, or other soy product)

 Skim milk, buttermilk, evaporated skim milk, low-fat yogurt, low-fat cottage cheese, calcium-fortified soy milk, eggs such as Eggland's Best Eggs that are rich in omega-3 fatty acids (100 mg per egg), ricotta cheese (fat free)

½ **Edamame, garbanzo, pinto, kidney, black, lima, or white beans; split, black-eyed, or field peas; lentils**

  Parmigiano-Reggiano, grana padana, string cheese, Neufchâtel (reduced-fat cream cheese), soy cheese, peanut butter, almond butter or other nut butters, walnuts, almonds, Brazil nuts, cashews, chestnuts, hazelnuts, macadamia nuts, mixed nuts, peanuts, pecans, pine nuts, pistachios, soy nuts, pumpkin seeds, sunflower seeds

 Swiss, Cheddar, mozzarella, Romano, colby, feta, Gorgonzola, goat, or Monterey Jack cheese

Carbohydrate Sources

Grain products enriched with folate, such as: whole grain bread, corn tortilla, whole wheat tortilla, whole grain English muffin or bagel, focaccia bread, whole wheat pita or ½ round whole grain lavash, whole grain crackers, corn bread, polenta, whole grain muffins, whole grain waffles, or pancakes

Popped popcorn

High-fiber cereal, muesli enriched with folate

Apple, banana, berries, carambola (star fruit), cherries, citrus, grapes, kiwifruit, melon, mango, nectarine, peach, pear, pineapple, plum

100% fruit juice, plain or calcium-fortified (limit to once a day)

½ Grain products enriched with folic acid such as: grits, oatmeal, Wheatena; couscous; whole wheat pasta, pasta with at least 2 grams of fiber per serving; brown rice or other whole grain; garbanzo, pinto, kidney, black, lima, or white beans; split, black-eyed, or field peas; lentils; edamame; corn; green peas; potatoes with skin; acorn or butternut squash; sweet potatoes or yams; plantain

> Check out the *Freebie* list for lots of veggies, including salad greens, tomatoes, carrots, etc., that you don't have to limit.

Dried fruit such as raisins, cherries, blueberries, apricots, plums, figs, etc.

Flaxseed meal, wheat germ

Fat Sources

MONOUNSATURATED FATS

Avocado, **olives,** hummus, almonds, Brazil nuts, cashews, chestnuts, hazelnuts, macadamia nuts, mixed nuts, peanuts, pecans, pine nuts, pistachios, **soy nuts, walnuts,** pumpkin seeds, safflower seeds, sesame seeds, sunflower seeds

🖐 **Olive oil, canola oil,** peanut oil, tahini paste, low–trans fat margarines such as Olivio

Polyunsaturated Fats

🖐 🖐 Benecol Light or Take Control Light spread, salad dressing, light margarine, light mayonnaise, light salad dressing, and low–trans fat margarines such as Smart Balance

🖐 Benecol or Take Control spread, corn oil, safflower oil, soybean oil, sesame oil, sunflower oil, tartar sauce, salad dressing

Freebies

Beverages: Coffee, tea, or diet caffeinated soft drinks up to caffeine limits of 600 mg a day. Once your caffeine limit is met for the day, decaf coffee, decaf tea—or caffeine-free diet soft drinks, club soda, carbonated or mineral water

Veggies: Artichoke, artichoke hearts, arugula, asparagus, bean sprouts, beets, Bibb lettuce, broccoli, Brussels sprouts, carrots, cauliflower, cabbage, celery, collard greens, cucumber, endive, eggplant, escarole, green beans, green onions or scallions, green, red, or yellow pepper, kale, kohlrabi, leeks, lettuce, mixed greens, mesclun, mushrooms, mustard greens, okra, onions, pea pods, radishes, romaine, spinach, summer squash, tomato, turnips, turnip greens, water chestnuts, zucchini

Miscellaneous: Broth or bouillon, ketchup, horseradish, lemon juice, lime juice, mustard, pickles, soy sauce, taco sauce, salsa, vinegars, garlic, fresh or dried herbs, pimento, spices, wine used in cooking, Worcestershire sauce, sugar substitutes

Sweets, Treats, and Alcohol

The Phenotype A Diet allows you two fists 👊 👊 to use as you desire, within some limits. If you are a recovering alcoholic, you obviously can't use your two fists on alcohol. If your trigger food is pizza, it isn't a good idea to indulge in pizza. So choose your two fists of treats from foods other than your trigger foods or your former addictive substances. To use the two fists 👊 👊 as treats, you don't have to subtract anything from the

Phenotype A Diet. These calories were already included in the calculations. Remember to include everything you eat in your Food Record.

To use the two fists 👊 👊 as treats, you don't have to subtract anything from the Phenotype A Diet.

SAMPLE MENUS

On days when you're rushed, use the NO-TIME Menus. MORE-TIME Menus are for days when you can cook leisurely. The menus are also meant to serve as a guide for eating out.

NO-TIME Menu A for Women

MEAL 1

Sliced French baguette with:

👊 👊 Natural peanut butter **or** Swiss cheese

Fresh peach

Freebie beverages

MEAL 2

Roasted turkey sandwich with:

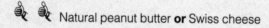 Hearty oatmeal bread

Freebie Sliced plum tomato

Freebie Red or green leaf lettuce leaves

👊 👊 Sliced avocado

Freebie Honey and Dill Mustard (such as Harry and David's)

Freebie Baby carrots

Freebie Evian or other favorite water

SNACK 1

 Cappuccino made with 1% milk

MEAL 3

Mexican black bean burrito with:

 Whole wheat flour tortilla

½ Black beans

½ Yellow corn

Freebie Salsa

  Shredded Mexican cheese (such as Sargento Reduced-Fat Mexican)

Freebie Spring salad mix with Balsamic-Dill Vinaigrette (see NO-TIME Recipes in Appendix C for dressing recipe)

Freebie beverages

SNACK 2

 Multigrain Cheerios

 1% milk/soy milk

MORE-TIME Menu A for Women

MEAL 1

 Poached egg (such as Eggland's Best)

 Pumpernickel-rye swirl bread with margarine (low–trans fat, such as Olivio)

 Watermelon wedge

Coffee and *Freebie* beverages

Meal 2

 Risotto with *Freebie* asparagus and lemon

Tomato, fresh mozzarella and basil salad (Caprese) with:

> *Freebie* Sliced tomato

>   Fresh mozzarella cheese

> *Freebie* Fresh basil

> Olive oil and *Freebie* balsamic vinegar

Freebie Iced decaf green tea or flavored water

Snack 1

 Low-fat yogurt (such as Stonyfield Banilla, a banana-vanilla mix) with:

>   Toasted walnuts

> Sliced fresh pear

Freebie beverages

Meal 3

Tuscan pasta salad with:

> Canned tuna (in water)

> ½ Garbanzo beans

> Whole wheat pasta spirals

> *Freebie* Chopped scallion

>   Black olives, sliced

> *Freebie* Chopped broccoli

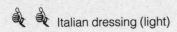 Italian dressing (light)

Freebie beverages

SNACK 2

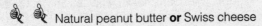 Popcorn, popped with light olive oil and sprinkled with freshly grated Parmigiano-Reggiano cheese

Freebie beverages

NO-TIME Menu A for Men

MEAL 1

Sliced French baguette with:

Natural peanut butter **or** Swiss cheese

Fresh peach

Freebie beverages

MEAL 2

Roasted turkey sandwich with:

Hearty oatmeal bread

Freebie Sliced plum tomato

Freebie Red or green leaf lettuce leaves

Sliced avocado

Freebie Honey and Dill Mustard (such as Harry and David's)

Red grapes, seedless

Freebie Baby carrots

Freebie Evian or other favorite water

SNACK 1

& ½ Cappuccino made with 1% milk or soymilk

MEAL 3

Mexican black bean burritos with:

Whole wheat flour tortillas

Black beans

Yellow corn

Freebie Salsa

Shredded Mexican cheese (such as Sargento Reduced Fat Mexican)

Freebie Spring salad mix with Balsamic-Dill Vinaigrette (see NO-TIME Recipes in Appendix C for dressing recipe)

Freebie beverages

SNACK 2

Multigrain Cheerios

1% milk or soy milk

MORE-TIME Menu A for Men

MEAL 1

Eggland's Best Egg

Pumpernickel-rye swirl bread with margarine (low–trans fat, such as Olivio)

Watermelon wedge

MEAL 2

 & ½ Risotto with *Freebie* asparagus and lemon

Tomato, fresh mozzarella and basil salad (Caprese) with:

> *Freebie* Sliced tomato
>
>   Fresh mozzarella cheese
>
> *Freebie* Fresh basil
>
> Olive oil and *Freebie* balsamic vinegar

 7-grain roll

Freebie Iced decaf green tea or flavored water

SNACK 1

 Low-fat yogurt (such as Stonyfield Banilla, a banana-vanilla mix) with:

>   Toasted walnuts
>
> Sliced fresh pear
>
> Fresh blackberries

MEAL 3

Tuscan pasta salad with:

> Canned tuna (in water)
>
> Garbanzo beans
>
> Whole wheat pasta spirals
>
> *Freebie* Chopped scallion
>
> Black olives, sliced

Freebie Chopped broccoli

👍 👍 Freshly grated grana padana cheese

👍 👍 Italian dressing (light)

✊ Mango cubes

Freebie beverages

SNACK 2

✊ ✊ ✊ Popcorn, popped with 👍 light olive oil and sprinkled with 👍 👍 freshly grated Parmesan cheese

Freebie beverages

Supplements

FOR DEPRESSION

St. John's wort (Hypericum perforatum): One of the most popular herbal remedies in the United States, St. John's wort is used to treat mild depression and anxiety. It is hence a natural choice for Phenotype As. However, if you presently take St. John's wort or are considering it, we have several caveats. Few people can accurately judge whether their depression is mild, moderate, or severe. If you are feeling depressed, before you try to self-medicate, it's important to see your physician or a licensed mental health professional for an assessment and recommendations. The most successful treatment for depression is *usually* a combination of talk therapy and medication. Neither works as well alone. If your depression is diagnosed as being in the mild category, ask about trying St. John's wort.

Purchase a St. John's wort supplement with its active compounds, the reddish pigment hypericin, and flavonoids from the flowers and leaves. Do not mix St. John's wort with prescription medications unless approved by your physician, because St. John's wort activates liver enzymes that metabolize drugs. Also, St. John's wort may reduce the effectiveness of medications such as protease inhibitors, cyclosporine, digoxin, warfarin, chemotherapy, antipsychotics, cholesterol-lowering agents, and theophylline. If you are already taking antidepressants such as monoamine oxidase inhibitors (MAOIs), selective serotonin reuptake inhibitors (SSRIs), other antidepressants, SAMe, valerian, or antimigraine medications, you should not take St. John's wort.

St. John's wort can also interfere with the absorption of iron and other minerals. In some cases it has caused breakthrough bleeding in women and rendered the birth control pill less effective. It's also important to note that St. John's wort can prolong the side effects of anesthesia, so be sure to let your doctor and anesthesiologist know about any supplements you are taking prior to surgery. Side effects may occasionally include fatigue, allergic skin reactions, headaches, or gastrointestinal complaints.

S-Adenosyl-L-Methionine (SAMe): This molecule occurs naturally in the body and is produced by a reaction between the amino acid methionine and adenosine triphosphate (ATP), a compound used by cells to perform all types of tasks. SAMe is involved in the production of the neurotransmitters (brain chemicals) serotonin, dopamine, and melatonin, which influence mood, and the components of cartilage, which support bone structure and strength. As a supplement, it is used for its antidepressant benefits and for osteoarthritis.

The cautionary note for St. John's wort applies to SAMe too. Before you try to self-medicate, discuss your condition and SAMe with your physician or a licensed mental health professional. As with St. John's wort, SAMe should not be combined with prescription antidepressants such as tricyclic antidepressants (TCAs), selective serotonin reuptake inhibitors (SSRIs) nor with monoamine oxidase inhibitors (MAOIs). If SAMe is taken, St. John's wort and/or valerian should not be used. Individuals with bipolar (manic-depressive) disorder should be aware that SAMe can trigger a manic phase.

Last, do not use SAMe if you are nursing or pregnant. Also, SAMe may be contraindicated for cardiac patients, since it can elevate homocysteine levels in the blood, a risk factor for heart disease. It may lower blood digoxin levels by up to 25 percent, so it is not recommended for cardiac patients who are using digoxin to strengthen their heart muscle contractions.

Omega-3 fatty acids: Omega-3 fats include eicosapentaenoic acid (EPA) and docosahexaenoic acid (DHA) and are common in the oils of fish. As mentioned in Focus Foods, they can also be made within your body from a precursor substance called alpha-linolenic acid (ALA) found in plant foods such as walnuts and flaxseed meal. Food sources of omega-3 fatty acids and ALA foods are included in your Focus Foods list. If you do not eat fish, fish oil supplements containing omega-3 fatty acids have been shown to have similar mood-stabilizing properties, triglyceride- and blood pressure–lowering effects, and anti-inflammatory effects, such as helping to prevent relapse in Crohn's disease or rheumatoid arthritis.

If you are a hemophiliac, taking prescription blood thinners such as warfarin (Coumadin) or heparin, or expecting to undergo surgery, fish oil supplements should be used only under a physician's care.

FOR POSTALCOHOL TREATMENT

Milk thistle (*Silybum marianum*): Milk thistle is an herb that has been suggested as an adjunctive treatment for diseases that negatively affect the liver, such as alcoholism, because it stimulates the liver to regenerate and form new liver cells. A blood test to check liver enzymes after four weeks of treatment is recommended to determine improvement.

B-complex vitamin: A B-complex vitamin is often used following alcohol treatment to replace the thiamine and other B vitamins lost during alcohol use. Excessive alcohol intake negatively affects the B vitamin thiamine in virtually every way. Thiamine is not converted to its usable, active form in the body when alcohol is present, and alcohol increases the loss of thiamine in the urine. In addition, people who consume large amounts of alcohol tend to get less thiamine from food. Moreover, their need for thiamine is increased because it is required to metabolize alcohol.

Phenotype A Maintenance

Phenotype A is the only diet that does not have a separate maintenance diet. That's because for Phenotype A, your goal is to focus on healthy eating and reduce, then eliminate, binge eating. The plan is designed to keep you doing that for the long term.

By getting rid of the calorie-intensive binges, you'll do away with the sources of your weight gain. You can shed your extra pounds and stabilize at your optimal weight. Remember Mary Ann? She started the Phenotype A Diet saying, "Binge eating is really what I'm all about." If you asked her now, she would say that following the Phenotype A Diet has given her back control of her eating. She'd tell you her turning point was the first month she went without a binge. She concentrated on changing her eating behaviors, didn't feel deprived on the Phenotype A Diet, and began to feel more positive about herself. She knew that from that day forward she could change for good. Impressively, Mary Ann hasn't had a binge in almost a year and she's in no way obsessing about her weight. She has lost weight and kept it off.

Some find that losing weight also allows them to change other things in their life that were making them unhappy. Positive changes in self-esteem, whether they come before or after weight loss, are critical to successful weight maintenance. Many of our clients have made positive changes in other aspects of their lives, such as starting a career, changing careers, finding a hobby or interest, or starting a relationship, and then felt ready to lose weight and keep it off. Regardless, long-term healthy eating, physical activity, and weight loss create a "feel-good" brain chemistry, whereas binge eating does not.

SUPPLEMENT
RECOMMENDATIONS AND DOSES

SUPPLEMENT	DOSE
ALL PHENOTYPE A:	
Multivitamin/mineral	Daily
Vitamin C	250 mg daily
Vitamin E	200 IU mixed tocopherols daily for women, 400 IU for men
FOR DEPRESSION:	
St. John's wort	2–4 g of the herb or the equivalent of 0.2 to 1.0 mg of total hypericin for four to six weeks and then evaluate for improvement; do not take if you are using valerian or SAMe
SAMe	400–1,600 mg per day in divided doses taken on an empty stomach about one hour before meals or two hours after meals; do not take if you are using valerian or St. John's wort
Omega-3 fatty acids	1–3 g per day in divided doses taken with meals
POSTALCOHOL TREATMENT:	
Milk thistle	200 mg twice a day containing at least 70% silymarin
B-complex vitamins	1 per day with food, not more than 200% of the daily value (DV) of each B vitamin included in the complex

The Phenotype B Diet

OUTSMARTING HIGH BLOOD
PRESSURE–LINKED WEIGHT GAIN

Bill's Story

"I was shocked at my last physical, when my blood pressure was 145/90."

Bill is a 28-year-old black man who married his high school sweetheart and is now the father of two young children. When Bill took our Phenotype Assessment, he didn't anticipate that he'd have genetic risk factors. "My mother had a stroke at age fifty-five, but she smoked two packs a day. I thought smoking caused her stroke so I never started," Bill said, adding that although his mom had never talked much about her blood pressure, after her stroke she revealed that it had always been high.

Bill had been the quarterback of his high school football team and was well known around his small town. When he finished high school, the young athlete played four more years on a college football scholarship. He majored in hotel and restaurant administration, and when he graduated he had no trouble getting a job as a restaurant manager back home. Working long hours and constantly being around food, Bill gained 25 pounds. "I didn't think I was eating too much. When I became a manager, I started drinking coffee and soft drinks and snacking during the day, but I also admit that I really piled it on at night. And with my schedule, I wasn't getting any exercise. Even so, I was shocked at my last physical, when my blood pressure was 145/90. My assessment indicated I was a Phenotype B, but I couldn't *believe it. Now I'm starting to think that my mom's high blood pressure is also a problem for me."*

If you're overweight and a Phenotype B, you answered "yes" to some of these statements in the Phenotype Assessment:

- My mother (or father) has or had high blood pressure or a stroke.
- My blood pressure typically runs above 120/80.
- I would describe myself as physically inactive.
- I drink more than 24 ounces of beer, 10 ounces of wine, or 2 ounces of liquor each day.
- I eat fewer than five fruit and/or vegetable servings a day.

STEP ONE: UNDERSTANDING YOUR PHENOTYPE

Phenotype Bs gain weight in association with a genetic tendency to high blood pressure, also called hypertension. If your blood pressure is edging above 120/80 and/or you or a family member has been diagnosed as at risk for hypertension, this is your phenotype. Research has established a strong connection between weight gain and harmful blood pressure levels, which are the leading cause of stroke, heart attack, and kidney disease. Interdependent, weight gain and high blood pressure both stem from a common genetic grouping that we call Phenotype B.

The Link Between Weight and Hypertension

The heart's job is to keep the blood pumping at optimum levels. Several factors contribute to hypertension, causing the heart to work harder, frequently to dangerous degrees. The most common source of hypertension is peripheral vascular resistance, which can be caused by plaque accumulation. *Arterioles,* small blood vessels that branch off from the arteries, become constricted with plaque, impeding the passage of blood. As a result, blood pressure rises, putting more demands on the heart. Increased blood volume due to fluid retention can raise arterial pressure even more, as can greater blood thickness, or "blood viscosity."

As Phenotype Bs overeat and gain weight, up goes their blood pressure. This is our clients' experience and probably yours as well, and it has been played out in numerous scientific studies, such as those published in *Obesity Research,* which associate abdominal fat (weight around the middle, also called visceral fat or android fat) with higher blood pressure. We have watched the rate of obesity in children rise together with the rate of high blood pressure. This underscores the genetic tie between high blood pressure and weight gain. Today, more than 350,000 American children have high blood pressure, and that number will rise unless children acquire the healthful habits that will help them outsmart their genes.

We know that outsmarting Phenotype B genes works because losing weight, and particularly abdominal fat, is the single most effective treatment for hypertension, as many studies have indicated. The effectiveness of weight reduction in decreasing blood pressure has been well documented in both mild and severe hypertension. For example, losing just 10 pounds lowered subjects' blood pressure and normalized blood lipids and glucose in the research Trial of Anti-Hypertensive Intervention. In addition, the greater the weight loss, the greater the blood pressure reduction.

Scientists are just beginning to understand *why* hypertension, even prehypertension (being at significant risk for developing high blood pressure), go hand in hand with weight gain in Phenotype Bs. When you, as a Phenotype B, put on a few pounds as a consequence of too much of the wrong foods or a sedentary lifestyle, fat cells stimulate your adrenal gland to release two hormones, *aldosterone* and *cortisol*. Aldosterone misregulates blood pressure, causing it to rise. Cortisol, the hormone released during stress, is another part of the weight gain equation. Studies indicate that excess cortisol leads to fat storage in the midsection or stomach region. Overweight Phenotype Bs have significantly higher cortisol levels, almost three times as high as people of average weight. Researchers theorize that as a person loses weight, the levels of adrenal-stimulating factors that the fat cells produce, such as aldosterone and cortisol, decline along with the amount of fat stored in cells.

Fluid retention is another Phenotype B symptom. By design, our blood and tissues accommodate fluid; however, blood vessel walls are limited in their capacity to expand. If we begin to retain more water than necessary, our fluid levels rise. The healthier the vessels, the more adaptable they are. When the vessel walls—inclusive of arteries, veins, and capillaries—begin to reach maximum expansion, blood pressure increases. This effect is magnified when arterial walls are compromised by other factors, for instance by plaque accumulation from eating saturated fats (which may also have a genetic basis).

What makes us retain too much water? Compounds called *electrolytes* are a major force in maintaining fluid balance in our bodies. An imbalance of electrolytes causes water to be drawn out of cells and into the blood, increasing blood pressure. The minerals sodium, chloride, potassium, magnesium, and calcium are all electrolytes, but they play different roles in regulating fluid retention. Sodium and chloride—both ingredients of salt—act as sponges, promoting fluid retention and increasing blood pressure. Potassium reduces the peripheral vascular resistance we mentioned

A TASTE FOR SALT

We learn the preference for salt, one of the four major taste categories, early in life. If you give an infant a salty water solution, it makes an unpleasant face. But as infants begin to eat baby foods, crackers, and other items with salt, they start to like the salty taste sensation. By adulthood, the typical person eats a lot of sodium, greater than 4–5 g (4,000–5,000 mg) every day, more than twice the recommended amount, two thirds of it from processed food and one third applied at the table. But, it is possible to reverse the taste preferences you acquired since birth. You can "reprogram" your taste buds to prefer less salt, using less over a period of time.

earlier. By dilating the arterioles, increasing the loss of sodium and water from the body, and stimulating the sodium-potassium pump, potassium decreases blood pressure. Magnesium is an inhibitor of smooth-muscle contraction and works as a vasodilator, so it decreases blood pressure too. Most important, calcium, magnesium, and potassium do not work in isolation to lower blood pressure, but they are effective when consumed in food. Studies prove that increasing the amounts of calcium, magnesium, and potassium from food sources and decreasing salt intake significantly reduced blood pressure.

This effect was substantiated by an important study, Dietary Approaches to Stop Hypertension (DASH). The DASH study found that the less sodium consumed, the greater the drop in blood pressure. The diet used in the study was, in addition to being low sodium, high in mineral-rich fresh fruits and vegetables and low in red meat (which reduced the intake of saturated fats and cholesterol, thereby reducing plaque accumulation). This combination diminished blood pressure levels in most participants but had the greatest effect in those with high blood pressure. It did not take long to achieve results. Participants felt lighter within days because they shed a lot of water weight. And within two weeks their blood pressure began descending.

Why? Two reasons. Getting rid of salt immediately "squeezes out those sodium and chloride sponges," taking pressure off the blood vessels. As fruits and vegetables have a diuretic effect, they too help eliminate excess fluid through urine. Blood pressure decreases in up to 73 percent of Phenotype Bs who consume less sodium in their diet and more potassium, calcium, and magnesium. That is why we have made sodium reduction and fresh fruits and vegetables components of our Phenotype B Diet. And note that weight loss lowers blood pressure substantially more than a low-sodium/high-mineral diet alone.

The Silent Killer

These blood pressure–affecting mechanisms are at work in all of us. However, even though hypertension affects 50 million Americans—many are unaware that they have high blood pressure. Worse, it can be a silent killer. Often it has no obvious symptoms until a heart attack or stroke occurs. You could have high blood pressure for months or years and not even know it. As your blood pressure rises, you might experience headaches or flushing in the face and yet not make the connection. Untreated hypertension can reduce life expectancy by ten to twenty years. That is why it is so important that all of us get our blood pressure checked at least once a year and, for Phenotype Bs, as often as suggested by your physician.

Doctors gauge your blood pressure by correlating two numbers, the systolic and diastolic measurements. The *systolic measurement* is the pressure of blood against your artery walls when the heart has just finished pumping (contracting). It is the first or top number of a blood pressure reading. The *diastolic measurement* is the pressure of blood against your artery walls between heartbeats, when the heart is relaxed and filling with blood. It is the second or bottom number in a blood pressure reading.

Although treatment doesn't typically begin until blood pressure is in the range between 120/80 and 139/89, if your blood pressure is above 120/80, you are considered prehypertensive. You are a Phenotype B, and it is time to act. Again, though the exact genes are yet to be determined, we do know that the propensity for high blood pressure will be evident in your family history; it begins with multiple genes or gene variations. One need only look at the number of children who have the condition for confirmation. In the journal *Pediatrics,* a study indicated that young people between the ages of 5 and 27 with a family history of hypertension had significantly higher

WHAT IS OPTIMAL BLOOD PRESSURE?

CLASSIFICATION	SYSTOLIC BLOOD PRESSURE	DIASTOLIC BLOOD PRESSURE
Optimal	Below 115	and below 75
Normal	Below 120	and below 80
Prehypertension	120–139	or 80–89
Hypertension	140 or higher	or 90 or higher

systolic blood pressures and greater increases in blood pressure over time than those with a negative family history. In a study from *The Journal of the American Medical Association (JAMA)*, groups shown to be especially at risk for high blood pressure included women, especially black women, and people over age 60. Men with hypertension outnumber women during young adulthood and early middle age, but hypertension rapidly increases in women after the age of menopause and they soon outnumber men. Our stressful, sedentary lives contribute to these skyrocketing statistics. Processed, high-fat, high-sodium food pumps the numbers too. It is as though these outside influences have homed in on their targets—the hypertension hot spots in our genetic destinies—and activate them and reactivate them. What we are saying is that you have a choice: weight loss and better food choices and behaviors can keep your genetic tendencies under control.

Even if you are already taking antihypertensive medication, the Phenotype B Diet is still life-altering. Health care professionals have witnessed a synergistic effect of weight loss in people using medication to lower blood pressure. In patients who lost weight and were taking a blood pressure medication, the blood pressure decrease was greater than those taking only the drug and not losing weight. Thus, weight loss can reduce the amount of drug that is necessary and in some cases eliminate the need for medication!

Sherry's story

"This is my diet for life."

"I never had high blood pressure, or so I thought until my early forties. Now I'm finding out that I probably had it during my thirties. I started taking birth control pills after my daughter was born. And I gained weight right around my middle, just like a beach ball. I used to work as a nurse on a general medicine floor and was always on my feet, walking around. But after my daughter was born, I quit work to stay home with her. I thought I'd stay active, which didn't happen, but I kept eating the same amount of food.

"When I tried the Phenotype B Diet, I guess I thought I would lose some weight and then go back to my old habits, but that didn't happen. Instead of soda, a water bottle is my constant companion. I cut out all the chips, soda, crackers, and cookies, and boy did my grocery bill go down. Now I spend that money on fresh stuff. I love going to the store and stocking up on whatever is fresh and in season. My dad always had a garden, and it makes me feel closer to him to experiment with different 'crops' just like he did! I use my hand as a constant reminder of portions and remind myself that my stomach is only as large as my fist. Why stuff it to balloon size? I really *like having a treat every week! I've lost twenty pounds and kept it off. This has become my diet for life. It is so easy."*

You can immediately see why a Phenotype B like Sherry would benefit from eating less meat and substituting more fruits and vegetables for high-calorie sodas and chips. We'll explain more about how these changes affect blood pressure and weight positively in the Focus Foods section in a few pages.

STEP TWO: KEEPING A FOOD RECORD

Now that you understand the role of fluid retention in your weight gain and blood pressure, you will appreciate the critical need to revolutionize your habits—and how changing your food choices can immediately give you more control over your genes. The next step on the Phenotype B Diet is to keep a Blood Pressure and Diuretic Food Record. List all the fruits and vegetables (Diuretic Foods from the Focus Foods) you eat on a daily basis. Aim for five to ten fruits and/or vegetables daily. Keep track of your blood pressure, writing it down once a week for the first month and then monthly thereafter. The Food Record will help you correlate your evolving eating and lifestyle habits to your weight, blood pressure, and health on a day-to-day basis. Please see the example on page 77 of a daily record.

You can have your blood pressure checked at any fire station or health care facility, or on one of the commercial machines in drug stores or grocery stores.

Danielle's Story

A story of tragedy and triumph that Danielle has lived to tell.

A mother of four children, Danielle had many headaches and did not think too much about them. "One night, the pain was so intense that I knew my body was telling me something was very wrong, and I woke my husband for help. By the time we arrived at the hospital I had a brain aneurysm." Only 44 years old, Danielle then suffered a stroke during surgery and was in a coma for more than thirty days. "When I woke up, I felt like an alien in a foreign world. I couldn't speak, write, or remember anything." For six months, Danielle stayed in the hospital for rehabilitation to relearn the basics of daily living.

"When I was able to finally go home, I had to be moved by a lift, turned frequently, and worked on by a physical therapist several times a week. We could not

BLOOD PRESSURE AND DIURETIC FOOD RECORD

Date/Day	Blood Pressure (at least weekly)	Diuretic Foods	Total Number/Day

have made it without the love and support of friends and family. They set up a schedule of cooking as well as caring for me.

"A year or so later, when one of my sons started at the community college, he encouraged me to go also. I had never gone to college and thought that maybe it would help my memory and focus. I attended for two years and was able to make Bs and Cs. More than the grades, I improved mentally. Even though I still suffer from short-term memory loss, I am 57 and alive today to enjoy my three grandbabies."

At 252 pounds, Danielle is battling the aftermath of her stroke and her weight. Since starting the Phenotype B Diet, she has lowered her blood pressure and started to swim four to five times per week with a trainer. Keeping a record has helped her tremendously, since short-term memory loss from the stroke affects her recall. By recording her progress, Danielle keeps on track. She has make real headway in changing the types of food that she eats and is rethinking her portion sizes. For Danielle, less meat and more fruits and vegetables are now part of her everyday life. Down 25 pounds, Danielle is thrilled with her changes and is making progress every day on continued weight loss and improved blood pressure and cholesterol readings.

STEP THREE: DEVELOPING POSITIVE NONFOOD WEIGHT LOSS TRIGGERS

Importantly, though you have inherited the full complement of high blood pressure and weight gain tendencies, it is your behaviors that have been provoking both. The Phenotype B Diet detailed in this chapter changes the three food-related negative triggers from the Weight Trigger Quiz into positive weight loss triggers: best food choices, structured meals, and portion control. To rein in the poor nonfood behaviors and reverse their effects, you need to develop new strategies for controlling stress, and you need to become more active, incorporating regular exercise into your life.

Bill, for example, was surprised to score seven out of ten questions in the "Stress" category. He was in a less-than-healthy routine at the restaurant and didn't realize how much the constant tension was affecting him. As you recall, he snacked during the day and kept going on coffee and soft drinks, only to overeat at night as a way to destress. Sherry, on the other hand, quit work to take care of her daughter, and her inactivity made "No Regular Exercise" and "Increasingly Sedentary Lifestyle" her main triggers.

Changing triggers is not as difficult as it sounds. Don't pressure yourself to become faultless overnight. Just identify deliberate changes you believe you can achieve and begin to work toward them. *The decision to change* is the important part. Going back to Sherry, she made a conscious decision to make two changes: to work out along with an exercise video each morning and to take her daughter for a walk in the stroller every day.

Your goals shouldn't end up like New Year's resolutions—the long list of best intentions that are bungled by the second week of January. Over-reaching is setting yourself up for failure. As we told Sherry, make one change at a time, letting it become a habit before you start the next change. It typically takes three to four weeks for a change to become part of your life. Once exercising in the morning becomes part of your routine, just like brushing your teeth, you will be ready to move on to the next change.

A reward system may help you change more willingly. Set nonfood incentives, and reward yourself as you progress. For instance, Danielle loves to shop with her girlfriends and keeps a list of clothes and accessories that she uses for rewards when she reaches another goal. She recently bought a new swimsuit when she started swimming four times a week. Take a look at these other strategies for turning off your greatest weight gain triggers.

Reduce Your Stress

Everything needs to be done faster, better, and more competitively these days. We live in an atmosphere guaranteed to raise everyone's blood pressure, the more so for those who have the genetic predisposition. As explained earlier, overweight Phenotype Bs tend to react to stress with even higher volumes of the stress hormone cortisol, which leads directly to midsection weight gain.

Stress is the number one reason people abandon their diet plan. Bill, as an example, had lost 10 pounds when his mother (another Phenotype B) died suddenly from a second stroke. He was devastated. The funeral and aftermath were really hard for him. He and his wife had to go through his mother's things, divide them up between Bill and his brother, and then sell her house. He called a month after the funeral and said, "I messed up," meaning that stress had made him deviate from his diet.

Bill didn't really "mess up"; his reaction was normal. Sometimes when stress hits, you find yourself going back to your old habits for several days or even several weeks, usually for comfort. It is never too late to turn this situation around. Remember that you eat at least three times a day, and every time is an opportunity to change your direction. Do not let a bad day or a bad week or two keep you from obtaining your goal.

Bill knew his overeating was a direct result of the stress from losing his mom. He also knew that she would not want him to go back to his old habits, especially not because of her. So he went back on his diet and has now maintained his weight loss for three years.

Knowing that trying times affect almost everyone is all the more reason to develop some positive strategies to help you deal with stress each and every day!

- Go back to the plan if stress leads to a relapse. Adjust your attitude from "I blew the diet" to "One mistake is not a big problem—I am committed to this diet and losing weight with this diet." In order to lose the amount of weight you want to lose, you have to stay with your plan.
- Make eating a conscious and deliberate event, not something you do when you're stressed. You're less likely to feel satisfied and more likely to overindulge if you eat while driving, watching TV, working at the computer, or doing other activities.
- Write down what and when you stress-eat so you can become more accountable and conceive of different control strategies.
- Set aside a regular worry time. When stress tempts you to overeat or keeps you awake, put the thoughts aside until your scheduled worry time. Do not worry and eat at the same time.
- Clear out your schedule, if you are overcommitted, so you can have more time for yourself. Sometimes just one or two quiet evenings at home can rejuvenate you and help you feel more organized and in control.

Develop an Active Lifestyle

Choosing to be active, rather than sitting around, has many of the same effects as exercise. All moves toward a less sedentary lifestyle will help reorient your genetic predilection for weight gain and your confidence in making important changes.

- Turn off the television or computer at least three nights a week and plan other activities. Bill, as an example, found that by forcing himself not to watch TV, he played outside more with his kids, took his dog for a long walk at night, or got a chore on his to-do list done.
- Take regular breaks to stretch and interrupt the pattern of sitting and eating, especially if you spend time at work sitting in front of a computer. Set a timer on your PDA or computer to remind you to get up and move. Get rid of any food around your computer.

When you take a break, do anything but head to the kitchen. Create a new pattern and break the old habit.

- Make appointments for physical activity in your calendar and keep them. Danielle found that booking time with a personal trainer made her exercise. Later, as she felt more fit, she also realized that she *enjoyed* swimming and found herself looking forward to, rather than dreading, her regular swim time.
- At work, walk to visit coworkers rather than calling or e-mailing them.
- Take the stairs instead of the elevator whenever you are in a safe situation to do so.
- Carry your own groceries and other heavy items when possible, to increase your strength, build your muscle mass, and increase your metabolism.

Exercise Regularly

For Phenotype Bs, exercise has many benefits, but four of the best are that it lowers blood pressure, increases metabolic rate, reduces stress, and decreases body fat. It also produces endorphins, brain chemicals that help improve mood. If you feel too tired to exercise, remember that being physically active actually gives you more energy. Remember to take a bottle of water with you when you are exercising. Water helps meet your increased fluid need and is a great alternative to calorie-filled sports drinks or soft drinks.

- Use exercise as one of your enjoyable distractions when you have the urge to eat. Buy an inexpensive pedometer (order online from sites such as www.digiwalker.com and www.accusplit.com), and start counting your steps. This is an easy change because it increases motivation at the same time it increases exercise. Sherry found that just knowing how many steps she was taking as she pushed the stroller helped her think of other ways she could increase her activity. Challenge yourself to increase your steps by at least 100 every day until you reach your goal. You'll be surprised how motivating it is. Some pedometers even show how many calories you are burning!
- Find a walking or other activity partner and make dates to exercise together. Bill started playing tennis twice a week with a neighbor. It got him out of the house at night after dinner, and he was less likely to stay late at the restaurant, knowing he would disappoint his friend.

- Put exercise equipment in front of the TV set, so when you do watch TV, you can get some exercise while watching your favorite show.
- Commit to a short ten-minute walk, and you'll find it easier to keep going once you start. Walk around the mall at least once before you start shopping. Danielle found that she could do this with her girlfriends and work up her total steps to her goal of 10,000 steps (5 miles) per day. For Danielle, this amount included not just the exercise program but all Danielle's steps. It meant putting her pedometer on in the morning and wearing it all day. Try listening to a book on tape while you walk.

For many of you, these changes can easily be made on your own. But we know that for some of you these may seem like dramatic or even impossible changes. Because of their importance in changing your gene-based risks, please don't hesitate to seek help from a professional, such as a registered dietitian, licensed mental health professional, physician, or certified personal trainer.

STEP FOUR: FOLLOWING THE PHENOTYPE B DIET

The Phenotype B Diet helps you lose your unwanted weight and stop feeding your genetic predisposition for hypertension. You will replace a sodium-laden diet with one rich in calcium, magnesium, and potassium to lower your blood pressure. Significantly increasing your intake of plant-based foods will minimize fluid retention. Thus, the diet turns your food-based weight gain triggers into weight loss triggers with a specific food list, structured meals, and sensible portions. You will no longer be reinforcing the "silent killer" within you. This plan will change the person you are on a cellular level and ensure you a much healthier future.

The Phenotype B Diet will change your diet to lose weight and lower blood pressure with the following critical changes:

- The right balance of protein and plant foods
- A diuretic effect produced by food
- Reduced processed food and sodium intake
- Increased intake of potassium, magnesium, and calcium

Focus Foods

Phenotype B Focus Foods should become an integral part of your daily and overall eating plan, as they will facilitate weight loss while helping prevent and treat high blood pressure. They get you away from processed foods, which may be elevating your blood pressure. Besides their blood pressure–lowering benefits, these Focus Foods contain antioxidants and phytochemicals, naturally occurring substances that have health value way beyond basic nutrition.

By combining several of the Focus Foods, it may be possible to achieve a greater blood pressure–lowering effect than with one alone. We've included them in your Sample Menus and want you to make sure to add them into your diet on a daily basis. All of these foods can be eaten in conjunction with hypertensive medications.

Diuretic foods: Many fruits and vegetables have a very high water content that gives them a mild diuretic effect. Including those listed below in your diet may even diminish your need for diuretic medications, as was discovered in the DASH studies. In addition, naturally diuretic foods contain dietary fiber, which delays stomach emptying and keeps you feeling full longer.

    Diuretic fruits and vegetables: Apple, asparagus, banana, blackberries, blueberries, broccoli, Brussels sprouts, cantaloupe, carambola (star fruit), cabbage, carrots, cauliflower, celery, cherries, cucumber, endive, grapefruit, grapes, green beans, lettuces, mushrooms, okra, onions, orange, peppers, pineapple, squash, spinach, tomato, watermelon

Low-sodium foods: The suggested daily intake of sodium is around 2,400–4,000 mg. Sodium adds up quickly. The Phenotype B Diet reduces your sodium intake to 2,400–4,000 mg/day, which is the equivalent of 1 to 1½ teaspoons of salt, by allowing specific foods and disallowing others. Remember, two thirds of your sodium probably comes from processed foods and one third from salt added at the table. Read nutrition labels carefully and tabulate milligrams (mg). Obviously, lowering your intake of processed foods and not adding salt when you eat can have a dramatic effect on your blood pressure. You'll also feel less bloated from fluid retention.

Sodium Facts: What Does the Label Mean?

Label Description	What It Means in Terms of Sodium Levels
Sodium free or salt free	Less than 5 mg per serving
Very low sodium	35 mg or less of sodium per serving
Low sodium	140 mg or less of sodium per serving
Reduced or less sodium	At least 25% less sodium than the regular version
Light in sodium	50% less sodium than the regular version
Unsalted or no salt added	No salt added to the product during processing

Generally, the more processed a food is, the higher its salt content. So focus on fresh, frozen, and unsalted or low-sodium canned fruits and vegetables, low-fat milk products, and fresh lean meat and seafood. As you follow the Phenotype B Diet, you will see a decrease in your sodium intake as you replace processed foods with less processed ones.

When you cut your sodium intake, your food will initially taste a bit bland because your taste buds expect a certain level of sodium. However, the switch will be less noticeable if you replace salt and sodium with fresh herbs and spices and lemon or lime juice. Truly, your taste buds will adjust to be satisfied with lower levels of salt. And this will happen more quickly than you think—usually within a few weeks. Watching your blood pressure come down and feeling less bloated will make the adjustment easier.

Calcium foods (milk, yogurt, cheese): Calcium-rich foods such as dairy products can help you reduce your blood pressure and lose weight at the same time, as numerous studies confirm. The reverse is also true: other studies have reported that people who consume less calcium in food tend to be overweight and have higher blood pressure.

Fully 90 percent of women and 70 percent of men do not achieve the recommended calcium intake per day, which for Phenotype Bs is between 1,200 and 1,600 mg daily. One thousand mg is the average calcium intake for men, and 600 mg is the average for women, for whom calcium is extremely important to maintain bone density and strength. Studies associate each 300 mg daily intake of calcium (for example, 1 cup of low-fat yogurt) with about 6 pounds less weight in adults. And when two people consumed the same number of calories in a day, the person who consumed 1,000 mg of calcium from dairy foods lost more weight and fat than the one who consumed only 600 mg. As mentioned, calcium is an important electrolyte, helping to maintain a healthful balance of fluids in your system. In addition, high-calcium diets inhibit *lipogenesis,* fat-producing gene expression, and accelerate *lipolysis,* the breakdown of stored fat. By increasing the metabolic rate (the rate at which calories are burned), they further reverse fat storage and prevent weight gain.

The Journal of Nutrition attributes the hypertension benefits of milk products to the *combined* minerals potassium, calcium, and magnesium found in dairy products. Dairy products are also typically low in sodium, so substituting them for higher-sodium foods further lowers blood pressure.

Calcium from supplements, however, has not been shown to lead to weight loss. Further, excess calcium supplements can interfere with magnesium absorption, and magnesium is essential to reduction of high blood pressure.

Adding dairy foods to your diet is easy with all of the prepackaged yogurt smoothies, cheese sticks, and flavored milks in the grocery stores, or try a latte with skim milk for your midmorning coffee. In addition to dairy sources of calcium, soy products with calcium, orange juice and breakfast cereals fortified with calcium, and sardines and canned salmon with bones are good selections.

Magnesium-rich foods: Adequate supplies of magnesium in your diet will lower your blood pressure because it is a vasodilator. Refined carbs such as crackers, chips, and cookies lose up to 80 percent of their magnesium content in processing, so if you rely on highly processed foods, your magnesium intake will be inadequate. To boost your intake of magnesium in food sources, choose whole grains, spinach, potatoes, cheese, yogurt, almonds, cashews, peanuts, lima beans, black beans, black-eyed peas, oysters, strawberries, and bananas.

Potassium-rich foods: According to new and as yet not clearly understood findings, potassium has an even greater effect on blood pressure than calcium or magnesium, though again it is the *combination* of the minerals in *fresh* fruits and vegetables that produces the greatest benefit. Processed foods contain relatively low levels of potassium, as they do magnesium, so if you rely on them, you will not get enough potassium in your diet. In general, the more processed a food is, the lower the potassium content. That is another reason it's so important to become a label sleuth. *Fresh* fruits and vegetables, especially potatoes, kidney beans, spinach, melons, celery, orange and tomato juice, and bananas are good sources of potassium. *Fresh* meat, milk, yogurt, coffee, and tea also contain significant amounts of potassium.

Beans, seeds, and unsalted nuts: These foods bring fiber as well as magnesium, potassium, and zinc to the diet. Dietary fiber is helpful for weight loss in that it provides a feeling of fullness without adding substantial calories. Don't forget, those minerals have a powerful effect on blood pressure.

FOCUS FOOD FREQUENCY

FOOD ITEM	FREQUENCY
Diuretic foods	5–10 servings daily
Low-sodium foods	Daily
Dairy foods (low-fat or fat free)	2–3 servings daily
Magnesium food sources	Daily
Potassium food sources	Daily
Beans, seeds, and unsalted nuts	4–5 times per week

Begin with the Phenotype B *FAST TRACK* Two Weeks

With its quick results, the *FAST TRACK* Two Weeks gets you motivated to keep going. The *FAST TRACK* is too severe for achieving long-term changes to your phenotype, but it will jump-start your weight loss. You'll begin to feel leaner, healthier, and sexier within days. It uses the same format as the Phenotype B Diets for men and women below, with the following exceptions:

1. Omit the number of proteins, carbohydrates and fats from the Phenotype B Diet, as **boldfaced** in parentheses in the Meals and Snacks below.
2. Omit the two fist-size 🖐 🖐 portions of "Sweets, Treats, and Alcohol" (see page 91) allowed each week.
3. Take a multivitamin/mineral supplement as well as the recommended additional vitamin C and vitamin E daily (see "Supplements" on page 98)
4. Start Week 3 with the full Phenotype B Diet.

THE PHENOTYPE B DIET FOR WOMEN

Select your foods for each meal and snack from the Food List on page 89. Sample Menus using foods that fit the diet are on page 92.

Meal 1
1 Protein (any fist, ½ fist, or thumb[s] selection)
3 Carbohydrates **(omit 1 carbohydrate for *FAST TRACK* Two Weeks)**
Freebie beverages

Meal 2
2 Proteins (1 palm **or** any 2: fist, ½ fist, or thumb[s] selections) **(omit 1 protein for *FAST TRACK* Two Weeks)**
3 Carbohydrates **(omit 1 carbohydrate for *FAST TRACK* Two Weeks)**
Freebie vegetables
2 Fats **(omit 1 fat for *FAST TRACK* Two Weeks)**
Freebie beverages

Meal 3
2 Proteins (any 2: fist, ½ fist, or thumb[s] selections)
3 Carbohydrates **(omit 1 carbohydrate for *FAST TRACK* Two Weeks)**
Freebie vegetables
2 Fats
Freebie beverages

Snack 1
1 Carbohydrate
Freebie beverages

THE PHENOTYPE B DIET FOR MEN

Select your foods for each meal and snack from the Food List on page 89. Sample menus using foods that fit the diet are on page 94.

Meal 1
1 Protein (any fist, ½ fist, or thumb[s] selection)
4 Carbohydrates **(omit 2 carbohydrates for *FAST TRACK* Two Weeks)**
1 Fat
Freebie beverages

Meal 2
2 Proteins (1 palm **or** any 2: fist, ½ fist, or thumb[s] selections) **(omit 1 protein for *FAST TRACK* Two Weeks)**
3 Carbohydrates
Freebie vegetables
2 Fats
Freebie beverages

Meal 3
2 Proteins (any 2: fist, ½ fist, or thumb[s] selections)
4 Carbohydrates **(omit 1 carbohydrate for *FAST TRACK* Two Weeks)**
Freebie vegetables
2 Fats
Freebie beverages

Snack 1
2 Carbohydrates

Stopped losing weight? Refer to "How to Deal with Plateaus" on page 28 and reboot your diet with another *FAST TRACK* Two Weeks.

FOOD LIST

Focus Foods are in **bold type.**

How much of each food should you eat? Use your hand as your guide. Eat the amount that you see; that is, the size of your fist, your palm, or your thumb.

 PALM

 FIST

 THUMB

Protein Sources

Seafood. **Poultry without skin, or lean cuts of meat such as loin, round, or cutlets of beef, pork, veal, venison, lamb, etc.; cook by steaming, sautéing, broiling, or grilling.** Meat alternative (tofu, tempeh, or other soy product)

Skim milk, buttermilk, evaporated skim milk, low-fat yogurt, low-fat cottage cheese, calcium-fortified soy milk, **eggs such as Eggland's Best Eggs, that are rich in omega-3 fatty acids (100 mg per egg), ricotta cheese (fat free)**

½ **Edamame, garbanzo, pinto, kidney, black, lima, or white beans; split, black-eyed, or field peas; lentils**

Parmigiano-Reggiano, grana padana, string cheese, Neufchâtel (reduced-fat cream cheese), soy cheese, **peanut butter, almond butter or other nut butters, walnuts, almonds, Brazil nuts, cashews, chestnuts, hazelnuts, macadamia nuts, mixed nuts, peanuts, pecans, pine nuts, pistachios, soy nuts, pumpkin seeds, sunflower seeds**

Swiss, Cheddar, mozzarella, Romano, colby, feta, Gorgonzola, goat, or Monterey Jack cheese

Carbohydrate Sources

Whole grain bread, corn tortilla, whole wheat tortilla, whole grain English muffin, bagel, whole wheat pita or ½ round whole grain lavash, whole grain crackers, polenta, focaccia bread, corn bread, whole grain muffins, whole grain waffles or pancakes

Popped popcorn

High-fiber cereal, muesli

Apple, banana, berries, carambola (star fruit), cherries, citrus, grapes, kiwi fruit, melon, mango, nectarine, peach, pear, pineapple, plum

100% fruit juice, plain or calcium-fortified (limit to once a day)

½   Grits; oatmeal; Wheatena; couscous; whole wheat pasta, pasta with at least 2 grams of fiber per serving; brown rice or other whole grain; **garbanzo, pinto, kidney, black, lima, or white beans; split, black-eyed, or field peas; lentils; edamame; corn; green peas; potatoes with skin; acorn or butternut squash; sweet potatoes or yams; plantain**

Dried fruit such as raisins, cherries, blueberries, apricots, plums, figs, etc.

Flaxseed meal, wheat germ

> Check out the *Freebie* list for lots of veggies, including salad greens, tomatoes, carrots, etc., that you don't have to limit.

Fat Sources

MONOUNSATURATED FATS

Avocado, olives, **hummus, almonds, Brazil nuts, cashews, chestnuts, hazelnuts, macadamia nuts, mixed nuts, peanuts, pecans, pine nuts, pistachios, soy nuts, walnuts, pumpkin seeds, safflower seeds, sesame seeds, sunflower seeds**

Olive oil, canola oil, peanut oil, tahini paste, low–trans fat margarines such as Olivio

Polyunsaturated Fats

🥄 🥄 Benecol Light or Take Control Light spread, light margarine, light mayonnaise, light salad dressing, low–trans fat margarine such as Smart Balance

🥄 Benecol or Take Control spread, corn oil, safflower oil, soybean oil, sesame oil, sunflower oil, tartar sauce, salad dressing

Freebies

Beverages: Coffee, tea, or diet soft drinks up to caffeine limit of 450 mg/day, club soda, carbonated or mineral water

Veggies: Artichoke, artichoke hearts, arugula, asparagus, bean sprouts, beets, Bibb lettuce, broccoli, Brussels sprouts, carrots, cauliflower, cabbage, celery, collard greens, cucumber, endive, eggplant, escarole, green beans, green onions or scallions, green, red, or yellow pepper, kale, kohlrabi, leeks, lettuce, mixed greens, mesclun, mushrooms, mustard greens, okra, onions, pea pods, radishes, romaine, spinach, summer squash, tomato, turnips, turnip greens, water chestnuts, zucchini

Miscellaneous: Broth or bouillon (low sodium), ketchup, horseradish, **lemon juice, lime juice,** mustard, soy sauce (reduced sodium), taco sauce, **salsa, vinegars, garlic, fresh or dried herbs, pimento, spices,** red wine used in cooking, Worcestershire sauce, sugar substitutes.

Sweets, Treats, and Alcohol

Okay, we know you're wondering, "Where are my treats like ice cream, my favorite red wine or a piece of chocolate toffee?" You'll be happy to know that we have designed this Phenotype B Diet to allow you two fists 🖑 🖑 per week to use as you desire. To use the two fists 🖑 🖑 as treats, you don't have to subtract anything from the Phenotype B Diet. These portions were already included in our calculations for your diet.

Red wines have particularly high levels of tannins, anthocyanins, and flavonoids, all members of the naturally occurring phytochemical family. These substances, found in greater concentrations in red wine than white, seem to be team players in preventing platelet activity, which can elevate blood pressure. Flavonols, the same substances found in red wine, are also in chocolate. Flavonoids aid blood pressure by improving blood vessel function, specifically blood vessel dilation or elasticity.

Although chocolate is high in fat, about one third of the fat is stearic acid, which doesn't cause an increase in your blood cholesterol. Cocoa powder and chocolate also add trace minerals to the diet, such as magnesium, copper, and potassium. You could splurge on your favorite chocolate such as Godiva or Dove. Currently, Dove Dark Chocolates contain a flavonol-rich chocolate called Cocoapro that is being used in a number of studies. How's that for some good news? Or maybe pull out all the stops and send for treats from Chocolat Debauve & Gallais on the Rue des Saints-Pères in Paris—whatever delights and satisfies your passion for good chocolate. That's the beauty of it—it's your choice. By allowing alcohol and treats, you're much less likely to feel deprived and want to overeat.

> To use the two fists as treats, you don't have to subtract anything from the Phenotype B Diet.

SAMPLE MENUS

On days when you're rushed, use the NO-TIME Menus. MORE-TIME Menus are for days when you can cook leisurely. The menus are also meant to serve as a guide for eating out.

NO-TIME Menu B for Women

MEAL 1

 Lemon Squeezer smoothie

   1 banana
   1 cup frozen raspberries
   ½ cup low-fat vanilla frozen yogurt
   ½ cup lemon sherbet

Place all ingredients into a blender or food processor. Blend thoroughly.

or

Go to a smoothie bar and order a *small* one with similar ingredients.

Freebie beverages

> Commercial smoothies are typically packed with calories, so order the small size. Forgo the add-ons, such as protein powder, herbs, and other supplements. Try to match your ingredients with those of your diet plan.

MEAL 2

🐚 Cheddar and Zucchini Bruschette (see this NO-TIME Recipe in Appendix C)

✊ ✊ Cherry-Banana Toss with 🥄 Orange Italian Dressing (see NO-TIME Recipes in Appendix C)

Freebie vegetables

Iced tea with a lemon slice or other *Freebie* beverages

MEAL 3

🐚 Classic Salmon with ✊ Confetti Vegetables (see NO-TIME Recipes in Appendix C)

½ ✊ Steamed brown rice (can also use quick-cook microwave brown rice)

✊ Grapefruit and Kiwi Salad with 🥄 Poppy Seed Dressing (see NO-TIME Recipes in Appendix C)

San Pellegrino sparkling water or other *Freebie* beverages

SNACK 1

 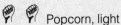 Popcorn, light

MORE-TIME Menu B for Women

MEAL 1

✊ Omelet with *Freebie* diced red, green, or yellow pepper and onions

½ ✊ Cinnamon-Applesauce Muffins (see MORE-TIME Recipes in Appendix C)

✊ Fresh blueberries and strawberries

Hot green, black, or oolong tea, or other *Freebie* beverages

MEAL 2

Carrot Chowder with Turkey (see MORE-TIME Recipes in Appendix C)

Pumpernickel-rye swirl bread

Freebie vegetables

Hot oolong tea with lemon or other *Freebie* beverages

MEAL 3

Garlic-Crusted Chicken with Pecorino Romano Cheese (see MORE-TIME Recipes in Appendix C)

Baked sweet potato

Zesty Green Beans (see NO-TIME Recipes in Appendix C)

Freebie vegetables

Lime-infused sparkling water or other *Freebie* beverages

SNACK 1

Zucchini bread

NO-TIME Menu B for Men

MEAL 1

1½ Lemon Squeezer smoothie

  1 banana
  1 cup frozen raspberries
  ½ cup low-fat vanilla frozen yogurt
  ½ cup lemon sherbet

  Place all ingredients into a blender or food processor. Blend thoroughly.

or

Go to a smoothie bar and order a *small* one with similar ingredients.

Commercial smoothies are typically packed with calories, so order the small size. Forgo the add-ons, such as protein powder, herbs, and other supplements. Try to match your ingredients with those of your diet plan.

Freebie beverages

MEAL 2

Cheddar and Zucchini Bruschette (see NO-TIME Recipes in Appendix C)

Cherry-Banana Toss with Orange Italian Dressing (see NO-TIME Recipes in Appendix C)

Freebie vegetables

Iced tea with a lemon slice or other *Freeble* beverages

MEAL 3

Classic Salmon with Confetti Vegetables (see NO-TIME Recipes in Appendix C)

Steamed brown rice (can also use quick-cook microwave brown rice)

Grapefruit and Kiwi Salad with Poppy Seed Dressing (see NO-TIME Recipes in Appendix C)

San Pellegrino sparkling water or other *Freebie* beverages

SNACK 1

Popcorn, light

MORE-TIME Menu B for Men

MEAL 1

Omelet with *Freebie* diced red, green, or yellow pepper and onions

Cinnamon-Applesauce Muffins (see MORE-TIME Recipes in Appendix C)

Fresh blueberries and strawberries

Hot green, black, or oolong tea, or other *Freebie* beverages

MEAL 2

Carrot Chowder with Turkey (see MORE-TIME Recipes in Appendix C)

Pumpernickel-rye swirl bread

Freebie vegetables

Hot oolong tea with lemon or other *Freebie* beverages

MEAL 3

Garlic-Crusted Chicken with Pecorino Romano Cheese (see MORE-TIME Recipes in Appendix C)

Baked sweet potato

Zesty Green Beans (see NO-TIME Recipes in Appendix C)

Freebie vegetables

Lime-infused sparkling water or other *Freebie* beverages

SNACK 1

Zucchini bread

Supplements

Garlic: Garlic has a long legacy of health benefits. In addition to its antibacterial properties and ability to "clear the arteries," garlic supplements can lower blood pressure by 5 to 10 percent, according to studies. For the prehypertensive group without diagnosed high blood pressure, garlic may be a treatment option before blood pressure medications.

Garlic supplements require the enzyme alliinase to convert alliin to allicin, once the pill is swallowed and touches liquid. The problem with supplements is that this alliinase enzyme is destroyed by stomach acid, so the true availability of allicin is hard to quantify. Some garlic pills, such as Kwai, are enteric-coated to bypass stomach acid and remain intact until they get to the intestine. In these, the garlic odor is mostly eliminated and the therapeutic benefits are protected.

But the more we learn about medical nutrition therapy, the more we realize that there are many compounds in food that may be active in the body beyond the ones currently known. For example, the garlic supplement Kyolic Extract utilizes the ingredient *S*-allyl-cysteine (SAC) instead of allicin. If you are also taking aspirin, vitamin E, or another blood-thinning medication, ask your physician before beginning garlic supplements, since they also affect clotting time. Adding garlic to your diet as a Focus Food is a better choice if you are taking these medications.

Calcium: Calcium supplements have no proven benefit in lowering blood pressure by themselves, as mentioned in the "Focus Foods" section. However, if you already have hypertension, several studies indicate that calcium supplements can help you achieve the right balance of minerals.

Stevia: Best known as an herbal sweetener, the herb stevia has been shown to have antihypertensive effects. In a one-year study of hypertensive people, 250 milligrams (mg) of stevia taken three times a day reduced blood pressure by 10 percent after three months of use.

Coenzyme Q_{10}: Studies suggest that CoQ_{10} can lower blood pressure by about 10 percent. Due to its modest effect, CoQ_{10} works best in people with prehypertension.

SUPPLEMENT
RECOMMENDATIONS AND DOSES

SUPPLEMENT	DOSE
Multivitamin/mineral	Daily
Vitamin C	250–500 mg daily
Vitamin E	200 IU daily for women, 400 IU for men, preferably of mixed tocopherols
Enteric-coated garlic	900 mg daily if you don't use garlic in cooking
Calcium (citrate or carbonate)	1,200–1,600 mg daily in divided doses of not more than 500 mg each; Viactiv Soft Calcium Chews are a tasty way to get 500 mg of supplemental calcium
Stevia	250 mg three times a day
Coenzyme Q_{10}	60–120 mg daily

The Phenotype B Maintenance Diet

Remember when you started on the Phenotype B Diet? In a few days, something inside just seemed to click and you began to lose weight, feel better, and feel healthier. That will not change. When you reach your weight goal, you are ready to move on to the Phenotype B Maintenance Diet. The diet has the same backbone Focus Foods. Still tailored to your genetic blueprint, it will keep you satisfied and your weight constant. A high level of physical activity or exercise is the single best predictor of keeping lost weight off. So keep moving!

THE PHENOTYPE B
MAINTENANCE DIET FOR WOMEN

Meal 1
1 Protein (any fist, ½ fist, or thumb[s] selection)
3 Carbohydrates
1 Fat
Freebie beverages

Meal 2
2 Proteins (1 palm **or** any 2: fist, ½ fist, or thumb[s] selections)
3 Carbohydrates
Freebie vegetables
2 Fats
Freebie beverages

Meal 3
2 Proteins (any 2: fist, ½ fist, or thumb[s] selections)
4 Carbohydrates
Freebie vegetables
1 Fat
Freebie beverages

Snack 1
1 Carbohydrate
Freebie beverages

THE PHENOTYPE B
MAINTENANCE DIET FOR MEN

Meal 1
1 Protein (any fist, ½ fist, or thumb[s] selection)
4 Carbohydrates
1 Fat
Freebie beverages

Snack 1
2 Carbohydrates

Meal 2
2 Proteins (1 palm **or** any 2: fist, ½ fist, or thumb[s] selections)
4 Carbohydrates
Freebie vegetables
2 Fats
Freebie beverages

Meal 3
2 Proteins (any 2: fist, ½ fist, or thumb[s] selections)
4 Carbohydrates
Freebie vegetables
2 Fats
Freebie beverages

Snack 1
2 Carbohydrates
Freebie beverages

CHAPTER 6

The Phenotype C Diet

OUTSMARTING CARDIOVASCULAR
DISEASE—LINKED WEIGHT GAIN

Sarah's Story

"I don't want to end up like my dad, dead at 44."

Sarah retired after twenty-seven years in the Navy, where she had obviously loved her job in the JAG Corps. Fit and trim, she had regularly passed the physical fitness assessment with flying colors. "When I was young," she wrote in her journal, "I was always attracted to the military for their focus on fitness. I decided that the Navy was for me because I didn't want history to repeat itself. My dad dropped dead of a heart attack while mowing the yard, and he was only forty-four. My Mom was devastated. He was her life. I watched her suffer and felt guilty that I couldn't fix it. Two of Daddy's brothers also died of heart disease before age 50.

"After leaving the military, I went to work for a law firm specializing in government contracts. The hours are brutal, leaving little time for me. So here I am, five years later and fifty pounds heavier."

Weight and guilt are not the only issues facing Sarah at age 51. Her cholesterol level is way above normal, and her HDL (protective cholesterol) is low. Her triglycerides shot up to over 1,000 mg/dl (normal is less than 150 mg/dl). She is clearly a Phenotype C. Given the new cardio risk indicators, it is crucial for Sarah to lose weight and keep it off forever. More than family history is contributing to Sarah's risk factors; changing her eating and behaviors is key.

If you're overweight and a Phenotype C, you answered "yes" to some of these quiz statements in the Phenotype Assessment:

- My mother (or father) had a heart attack or was diagnosed with heart disease before age 65.
- My bad (LDL) cholesterol is **above** 100 mg/dl.
- My good (HDL) cholesterol level is **below** 45 mg/dl (for men) or 55 mg/dl (for women).
- I watch TV more than three hours a day or would describe my exercise level as inactive.
- I carry my excess weight predominantly around the waist as opposed to the hips.

STEP ONE: UNDERSTANDING YOUR PHENOTYPE

Phenotype Cs gain weight in connection with a genetic tendency for cardiovascular disease. If you tend to put on pounds around your middle and/or you or a family member has been diagnosed as at risk for heart disease, this is your phenotype. Research has established a strong connection between people with abdominal obesity or android fat—what's called the "apple shape"—and harmful cholesterol levels, together with the concurrent formation of arterial plaque. Weight gain is one problem. The rising risk of heart attacks and strokes is another. Interdependent, both stem from a common genetic grouping that we call Phenotype C.

The Link Between Weight and Heart Disease

Heart disease is the leading cause of death today, killing someone every 33 seconds. More than one million Americans will have a heart attack this year, and one third of them will die. One in three men can expect to develop heart disease before age 60. One in ten women will develop heart disease before age 60, but almost half of all men and women alive today will die from it.

Roughly two thirds of the Phenotype C syndrome is attributable to genetics and one third to eating and other behaviors that often lead to weight gain. Since the Nurses' Health Study found a 30 percent increase in the risk of cardiovascular disease with each 15-pound increase in weight, it stands to reason that losing weight will dramatically reduce your risk.

The Phenotype C population is a big one because the invitations to join are ubiquitous. Many modern foods work against you. Saturated fat and partially hydrogenated fat, or "trans fat," as it is called, are in practically every baked product on grocery shelves. Fast food is loaded with saturated fat and trans fat. By elevating people's LDL (low-density lipoprotein) cholesterol, these fats encourage the buildup of arterial plaque. This, in turn, clogs arteries. Highly processed American food is largely devoid of antioxidants and other phytochemicals that safeguard against heart disease. (See Focus Foods section below.) In addition, inactivity does nothing to raise HDL or lower LDL, and it can actually work against both. If your life is stressful, the risks compound. Moreover, influxes of the stress hormone cortisol also tend to deposit extra pounds around the middle, feeding the apple shape and the plaque-producing cycle.

WHAT ARE LDL AND HDL?

LDL stands for *low-density lipoprotein,* and it is the carrier for cholesterol in the blood. An elevated level of LDL, the damaging cholesterol, indicates that fat is being deposited in the arteries, increasing the risk of a heart attack. HDL stands for *high-density lipoprotein,* and it is the protective cholesterol. It is the particle in the blood that removes cholesterol from the arteries and takes it to the liver to be removed from the body. The higher the HDL level, the better. *Hyperlipidemia* is low HDL combined with elevated cholesterol, LDL, and triglycerides. People with hyperlipidemia have an increased risk of heart disease.

WHAT ARE TRIGLYCERIDES?

Triglycerides are the chemical form in which most fat exists in food as well as in the body. They are found in increased levels in the blood following the digestion of fats in the intestine but are also made in the body from other energy sources such as carbohydrates. Calories ingested in a meal and not used immediately by tissues are converted to triglycerides and transported to fat cells to be stored as a potential energy source in adipose tissue (fat stored in the body). Triglycerides are released from fat tissue to meet the body's needs for energy between meals. The level of triglycerides rises in some people when they consume excess calories from alcohol, refined carbohydrate, and fat, producing a condition called *dyslipidemia*. High levels of triglycerides increase the risk of a heart attack.

Your Genes and Heart Disease

Phenotype C is a challenge to understand because more than 25,000 genes are associated with heart disease risk. Today when your physician orders a lipid profile, it typically quantifies total cholesterol, LDL, HDL, and triglycerides. You may get a C-reactive protein (CRP) measure as well, as this is another predictor of heart disease. Other indicators of risk are becoming important.

As an example, fascinating new research is looking at the pattern of LDL particles in overweight people who suffer from hyperlipidemia. Some have elevated numbers of small dense LDL particles and respond very well to changes in dietary fat. Sarah is in this group. By reducing her saturated fat intake, she reduces the number of small dense LDL particles and decreases her risk. She also overcomes fat as her fate. Others have a different pattern of larger, less dense LDL particles. These particles may be more protective, because they are not as likely to adhere to artery walls. These two distinct genetic patterns with two different risks illustrate how important and dynamic the future of nutrigenomics is.

Risks Other Than Your Genes

But what about those individuals who have elevated cholesterol, LDL, and triglyceride levels or decreased HDL levels, with no genetic predisposition or family history? This is the nongenetic form of hyperlipidemia, and it affects roughly one third of the U.S. population. Here, lifestyle factors alone increase risk. It is important to note, however, that people with either the environmental or the genetic type of hyperlipidemia can successfully lose weight and keep it off following the Phenotype C Diet along with the recommendations for minimizing and managing their environmental risk factors.

In concert with LDL, low-grade inflammation can further damage arteries. Indeed, even though inflammation is the body's way of combating infection, it can also exacerbate heart disease. Here's how: Your cells produce *cytokines*, proteins that promote chronic low-grade inflammation in the body, including the arteries. This inflammation triggers platelet formation in the blood. The platelets stick together, augmenting the formation of arterial plaque in the coronary artery that could dislodge and cause a heart attack. A study reported in *The Journal of the American Medical Association* (*JAMA*) found that obese women with android fat had greater platelet activation, a marker of inflammation partly precipitated by their excess weight and, of course, a risk factor for heart disease.

C-reactive protein (CRP) is an indicator of inflammation levels. CRP can be measured by a blood test called the *high-sensitivity CRP test* (hs-

CRP test) and is recommended for those with a family history of heart disease (Phenotype C) even when blood cholesterol is normal. Based on recent studies published in *JAMA*, it is evident that when Phenotype Cs gain weight around their middles, it drives their CRP levels and inflammation higher. The higher the CRP level, the greater the risk of heart attack. Phenotype C Focus Foods, weight loss, and lifestyle changes can lead to lower CRP levels. Remember, fully one third of the cause of heart disease resides in the six weight gain triggers named in the Weight Trigger Quiz on page 19.

José's Story

"I don't like being overweight, but what can I do?"

"The way my job is, I mainly have access to fast foods, and I sit most of the day. I know there are healthier choices at fast-food restaurants, but once I'm tired and hungry, nutrition goes out the window. Whenever I do decide to stop, I'm usually starved because I push myself to keep going. So I order the same old double burger, fries, and soft drink. It tastes good, and I don't have to think. Besides, it's more expensive to eat healthy out."

José is a 47-year-old electrician who drives all day from job to job in his van. Every time Jose got in his truck to go to work, he was accustomed to reach for something to drink, typically starting his day with a mug of high-octane java. After that, he'd purchase something sugary, such as a soft drink or sports drink. Jose didn't realize how many calories he was getting just in liquids. (A regular twelve-ounce soft drink has nine to twelve teaspoons of sugar.) These drinks quenched his thirst but not his hunger. José grabbed lunch and dinner at his favorite fast-food restaurants and, after a twelve- or fifteen-hour day, went home to his easy chair to watch TV and eat a home-cooked, usually high-fat meal.

José's cholesterol, LDL, and triglycerides were still within normal range, but his 25-pound weight gain around the middle, lack of exercise, late-night eating, and fast-food diet were strong personal Phenotype C in-

> The average person consumes more than 100 pounds of sugar every year in all types of processed foods and drinks.

dicators. Most important, though, his unhealthy habits, not his genetic patterns, put him at risk. José will tell you that it's diets that cause him to gain weight. He's been on and off quick-fix starvation diets ever since he hit 30.

On these roller-coaster weight loss plans, he not only gained back the weight he lost, he added more each time.

José came to one of our seminars, then started the Phenotype C Diet. Packing a food cooler for his truck and planning snacks of dried fruit and nuts made a big difference in his food choices. He also substituted noncalorie drinks and sugarless gum for his sugary drinks. José could eat well on the road and have to stop only for bathroom breaks. This helped keep his temptations under control. He discovered that he liked the sandwiches, fruit, and yogurt drinks his wife packed better than fast food. "I feel more alert, and I love being thinner. So far, I've lost about twenty-three pounds, and I've saved money too."

STEP TWO: KEEPING A FOOD RECORD

As part of the phenotype-based program, keeping a Food Record will help you keep track of how changing your food choices, portions, and eating habits affects your health and weight. Just as the data that scientists log and analyze demonstrate the validity of their experiments, the records you'll make will underscore why you are succeeding. We promise you that you will see positive results.

Focus Foods, which are detailed a few pages later, are an important element of the Phenotype C Diet, so your first step is to keep a tally of the Focus Foods you consume each day for a month. As you follow the Phenotype C Diet, you'll see your intake of these critical foods increase. We also ask you to record if and when you "stress-eat." You'll read more about this in the following section. To begin, either make copies of the following record or reproduce it in a journal you purchase.

Focus Foods

Date: _____

Fruits:

   (List and tally the items consumed) _____

Vegetables:

   (List and tally the items consumed) _____

Herbs and spices:

   (List and tally the items consumed) _____

Tea (black, oolong, and green):

   (List and tally the items consumed) _____

Purple/red grapes/grape juice/red wine:

   (List and tally the items consumed) _____

Plant stanol/sterol products such as Take Control Light and
Benecol Light or Minute Maid Heart Wise juice:

   (List and tally the items consumed)   _____

Garlic:

   (Enter tally here) _____

Soy protein:

   (Enter tally here) _____

Nuts and seeds:

   (List and tally the items consumed) _____

Beans and legumes/oats/apples:

   (List and tally the items consumed) _____

Olive oil/olives/canola oil:

   (List and tally the items consumed) _____

Seafood:

   (Enter tally here) _____

TOTAL NUMBER OF FOCUS FOODS: _____

TODAY'S SUCCESSES:

_____

_____

Food Issues You Noticed Today (stress eating, skipping meals, craving, etc.)

Date:_____ Issue: _____

Ideas for Changing or Turning Around These Issues:

_____

_____

_____

_____

_____

Jay's Story

"It's been over five years since that corporate wellness program. I've lost 100 pounds, and I've kept it off."

Jay, a customer service rep, walked into the Phenotype C Diet class standing 5'8" and weighing 260 pounds. When it was his turn to share why he had come to the class and what he expected to get out of it, he quietly and politely told us, *"I got hepatitis when I was twenty-one, and it destroyed my liver. I ended up having a liver transplant. Over the years, I've allowed myself to develop some pretty lame habits. I often go all day without eating, don't feel like exercising, and don't really like fruit or vegetables."* Before the first session was over, he confessed, *"But I'm tired of being heavy and tired of people saying stuff to me. It's a mental thing—how you look at yourself. What you look like is how you feel, and I don't feel good about either."*

This is a common complaint among our overweight corporate students— particularly those whose sedentary work keeps them sitting in front of a computer for long hours. Our class resources include an audio CD to reinforce weekly lessons. Reviewing them, Jay realized that his poor eating and exercise habits were not only keeping him from losing weight, they could be causing severe problems with his liver and blood lipids, particularly cholesterol.

At the next class meeting, Jay proudly announced that he had added bananas to his diet. In fact, he'd eaten several during his first week and lost 10 pounds by the end of Week 3. We knew this guy was determined and ready to change. And change he did. By the end of the six-week corporate seminar series, he had added a few more fruits and tomatoes to his diet, he was taking the stairs instead of the elevator, and he was rarely seen at work without a bottle of water in his hands. Six months later, Jay had dropped a total of 50 pounds on the Phenotype C Diet.

But it didn't stop there. It's been more than five years, and Jay is still following the diet. He's taken 100 pounds off, and, more important, he's kept it off. "I stay between 150 and 160, and I walk a lot—between twenty minutes and two hours at a time—and I bike three times a week. Now I eat all kinds of fruit—mostly mixed fruit prepared in the store with pears, apples, oranges, melons, and pineapple. I also eat cucumbers, lettuce, tomatoes, carrots, and sometimes peas."

Jay explained how he had overcome setbacks and how the Phenotype C Diet had changed his life: "Since I have lost the weight, people treat me differently. The advice I would give is to do it for yourself and no one else. You really have to want it. There will be setbacks, but keep the faith in yourself and you can do it. People will say you can't, but don't listen. Believe in yourself, and you can do it. Start slowly and enjoy the process. If you try to rush it, you will get burned out. There's no quick fix, but give one hundred percent for only three weeks and you will feel better about yourself and feel better physically. Make sure you try some exercise after meals, like walking or biking around the block or playing with kids. Now that I have lost the weight, I feel better and can do more. It's changed my outlook on life and people."

STEP THREE: DEVELOPING POSITIVE NONFOOD WEIGHT LOSS TRIGGERS

Remember that when it comes to weight, your genetics and family history load the gun, but ultimately your routines pull the trigger—negatively, toward weight gain, or positively, toward weight loss. The Phenotype C Diet detailed in this chapter changes the three food-related negative triggers from the Weight Trigger Quiz into positive triggers: best food choices, structured meals, and portion control.

How did you score on the Weight Trigger Quiz's nonfood categories: "Stress," "No Regular Exercise," and "Increasingly Sedentary Lifestyle"? Because of her brutal hours at the law firm, Sarah answered true to eight out of ten questions in the "Increasingly Sedentary Lifestyle" category and six out of ten in the "Stress" category. Too much driving every day made "No Regular Exercise" José's main trigger.

When moving from negative to positive triggers in these categories, make deliberate changes, not perfection, your goal. As an example, even by substituting squeezing a rubber stress ball for sipping a sports drink, José gave himself an outlet for stress and cut his calories. One of José's other deliberate changes was to buy an inexpensive pedometer so he could track his steps daily. A positive trigger, exercise, empowered his phenotype, reinforcing his new eating habits with more efficient metabolism. When new triggers kick in and eating patterns change, weight loss happens easily. "I love my new 'toy' and feel naked without it," José said. "When I started, I was walking well under a thousand steps a day, and the goal of ten thousand seemed impossible. So I decided to try and increase my walking by two hundred steps a day. The first few weeks it was hard, but I'd clip on that pedometer every day anyway, and eventually walking became part of my daily routine. Now if I'm not close to ten thousand steps by the time I get home, I hit the pavement and take a walk after dinner!"

We recommend making one change at a time and letting it become a habit before you start the next change. It typically takes three to four weeks for a change to become part of your life. Set nonfood incentives, and reward yourself as you progress. Start a "wish list" of rewards to keep you motivated, and choose an item from the list every time one of your deliberate changes becomes part of your lifestyle—permanently. Have a look at these other strategies for turning off your greatest weight gain triggers.

Reduce Your Stress

Life today is stressful. Whether it's the lack of personal time, pressures on the job, or being sandwiched in by taking care of older parents and younger children, stress is ever present. Although some stress can be eliminated or controlled, some cannot. Stress is the number one cause of diet relapse (going off a diet plan). Moreover, stress affects Phenotype Cs in particular, because they are especially vulnerable to the around-the-middle fat storage that can be triggered by the stress hormone cortisol. So you need some positive strategies to help you deal with stress each and every day.

- Go back to the plan if stress leads to a relapse. Adjust your attitude from "I blew the diet" to "One mistake is not a big problem—I am committed to this diet and losing weight with this diet." In order to lose the amount of weight you want to lose, you have to stay with your plan.
- Set aside a regular worry time for problem solving. When stress tempts you to overeat or keeps you awake, put the thoughts aside until your scheduled worry time.
- Carve out time to destress. Sarah found that working out at the local YMCA first thing in the morning three days a week helped control her stress. It became a regular appointment—with herself—to literally "work out" her tensions. She listened to the morning news while working out rather than reading the paper at home. Now that the deliberate change has become a routine, Sarah never misses her Monday, Wednesday, and Friday appointments and goes every weekday when her schedule permits.
- Make eating a conscious and deliberate event, not something you do when you're stressed. If you eat while driving, watching TV, working at the computer, or doing other activities, you're less likely to feel satisfied and more likely to overindulge. You may not even be aware of what or how much you're eating.
- If you find that you are a stress eater, record what, how much, and when you stress-eat in your Food Record. Notice the stress patterns that affect what you eat, and choose Phenotype C Focus Foods instead when you're stressed. A soothing cup of green tea works wonders to calm your nerves.
- If you are overcommitted, clear out your schedule so you can have more time for yourself. Sometimes just one or two quiet evenings at home can rejuvenate you and help you feel more organized and in control.

Develop an Active Lifestyle

- Turn off the television or computer at least three nights a week and plan other activities.
- Take regular breaks to stretch and interrupt the pattern of sitting and eating, especially if you spend time at work sitting in front of a computer.
- Alter your typical routine to make it less sedentary. "I'm taking the stairs more often than the elevator," Jay told us after a few weeks on the Phenotype C Diet. "Sometimes when I just need to get away from the phone or the screen, I go down the back stairs,

around the building, and up the front stairs. My coworker Dan and I take short, brisk walks when we can. Sometimes they're meetings on the move; we can discuss things more easily when we're away from the usual interruptions, and we don't have to reserve a meeting room!"

- Set a timer on your PDA or computer to remind you to get up and move.
- Carry your own groceries and other heavy items when possible to increase your strength, build your muscle mass, and increase your metabolism.

Exercise Regularly

Exercise deflates stress, prevents boredom, and revs up metabolism for hours after the activity. It also produces endorphins, brain chemicals that help to improve mood. For Phenotype Cs, exercise lowers LDL levels and increases the positive HDL in the blood. As you may recall, Sarah had a low HDL level and high cholesterol, so regular and ongoing exercise was one of her deliberate changes. She now walks between floors at the law firm instead of taking the elevator. She also makes a point of parking farther away from the door when she attends government meetings—or, better yet, walks to the meeting if possible. These efforts count as frequent bouts of exercise.

- When you have the urge to eat, use exercise as one of your enjoyable distractions. Jay began to ride a bike again, something he had not done since he was young, and remembered how much he enjoyed it. During the week he takes short rides, and on weekends, he and several friends plan longer rides.
- Strap on a pedometer like José and challenge yourself to increase your steps everyday until you reach your goal. You can buy one inexpensively at sporting goods stores or order one online from sites such as www.digiwalker.com and www.accusplit.com. This easy change, one that all the phenotypes can make, increases motivation at the same time that it increases exercise. Set a goal to increase your distance by at least 100 steps each day. You'll be surprised how motivating it is. Some pedometers even show how many calories you are burning!

For many of you, these changes can easily be made on your own. But we know that for some of you these may seem like dramatic or even impossible changes. Because of their importance in changing your gene-based risks, please don't hesitate to seek help from a professional, such as a registered dietitian, licensed mental health professional, physician, or certified personal trainer.

STEP FOUR: FOLLOWING THE PHENOTYPE C DIET

The Phenotype C Diet cuts to the heart (no pun intended) of losing weight and reducing your risk of heart disease by turning your food-based weight triggers into weight loss triggers with a specific food list, structured meals, and sensible portions. This diet also works on a cellular level to decrease cardiovascular disease risk by improving your lipid profile. As a result, you will feel healthier and more energetic and avoid fat as your fate.

Focus Foods

Research has shown the following foods to be beneficial specifically to Phenotype Cs. They will help prevent and treat heart disease while you're losing weight. By combining several of the Focus Foods, it may be possible to achieve a greater cholesterol-lowering effect than with one alone. All of them can be used in conjunction with statin medications. They are critical to the diet's design and success.

The Phenotype C Diet will change your diet to lose weight with the following critical changes:

- Eating seafood meals at least two times per week
- Including anti-inflammatory (salicylic acid) fruits and vegetables daily
- Increasing omega-3 fats relative to omega-6 fats to reduce LDL levels and inflammation
- Eating more nuts for their role in satiety and lipid profile improvement
- Switching from processed carbohydrates to high-fiber carbohydrates
- Substituting nonhydrogenated, unsaturated fats such as olive oil or canola oil for saturated fats and trans (partially hydrogenated) fats
- Getting rid of as much trans (partially hydrogenated) and saturated fat as possible

Salicylic acid (SA) foods: A recent study in the *Journal of Clinical Pathology* states that vegetarians whose typical diet is rich in fruits and vegetables have high levels of salicylic acid (SA) in their blood. Found in varying amounts in fruit, vegetables, and even herbs and spices, salicylic acid is related to the composite that is in aspirin (acetylsalicylic acid, which converts to salicylic acid) and has a similar anti-inflammatory action. It inhibits the function of cyclooxygenase-2 (COX-2), an enzyme tied to inflammation. Though not a substitute for medication or other treatment, eight to ten servings of SA-rich fruits and vegetables per day are definitely beneficial.

Foods High in Salicylic Acid
Fruit: Cherries, cranberries, currants, dates, raisins, prunes, raspberries, pineapples, plums, strawberries, boysenberries, grapes, oranges, apricots, cantaloupe, blackberries, and blueberries
Vegetables: Tomato paste, sauce, and canned tomatoes, cucumber, okra, spinach, green peppers, radishes, zucchini, broccoli, chili peppers, sweet potato, squash
Herbs and spices: Cayenne, cinnamon, curry, mustard powder, oregano, rosemary, sage, turmeric, mint, ginger root, basil, nutmeg, celery powder or flakes, paprika, tarragon, thyme, black pepper, bay leaves

Tea (black, oolong, and green): Abundant in flavonoids, catechins, and other phytochemicals that act as antioxidants, black, green, and oolong teas (all derived from *Camellia sinensis*) also contain a compound called epigallocatechin gallate (EGCG). You may have heard about EGCG as a green tea extract included in some weight loss products that supposedly crank up your energy level and metabolism to burn fat. A U.S. Department of Agriculture (USDA) study reported in *The Journal of Nutrition* found that energy output increased by about 3 percent when five cups of oolong tea were consumed per day. It's still not clear as to whether these effects are from the EGCG, caffeine, a combination of the two, or even other compounds in tea. The health benefits from drinking tea are very positive due to the flavonoids, catechins, and other phytochemicals, and if you get a metabolic boost on the side, that's even better.

> Black, green, and oolong teas come from the leaves of the *Camellia sinesis* plant. Herbal teas are derived from various flowers, herbs, and roots, so they don't have the same health benefits.

Data from the Rotterdam Study, a population study of Dutch adults over 55, analyzed over time found that the risk of a heart attack was lower in daily tea drinkers (about 12 ounces per day) versus non–tea drinkers.

Phytochemicals are naturally occurring substances in fruits and vegetables that provide significant health benefits. Phytochemicals such as flavonoids, tannins, and anthocyanins lower what is called *cellular oxidative stress,* the breakdown and destruction of healthy body cells by free radicals. Acting like sunscreen, these antioxidants help protect and keep cells and tissue healthy. They both destroy free radicals and protect against their effects.

The results of the Dutch tea analysis are in keeping with other research suggesting that tea flavonoids may protect against heart disease. Tea flavonoids and other antioxidants may protect your heart by decreasing the probability of blood clots, improving blood vessel elasticity, and preventing LDL cholesterol damage by free radicals, which increases the chance of plaque buildup in the arteries.

Purple and red grapes and grape juice: As naturally occurring antioxidants, the flavonoids found in purple grapes and grape juice help reduce the risk of heart disease.

In a recent study by the University of Texas Southwestern Medical Center, researchers found that flavonoids in Concord grape juice provided antioxidant protection in the body similar to that of Vitamin E (alpha-tocopherol). Tannins, anthocyanins, and flavonoids—found in greater concentrations in red wine than white—inhibit platelet activity. The grapes used to make purple juice have many of the same phytochemicals found in red wine. Researchers suspect that drinking grape juice or red wine daily may have a cumulative effect and provide cardiovascular protection.

For all the benefits of wine, it and other alcoholic beverages can elevate your blood triglyceride level. If you have high triglycerides, it may be prudent to limit or even omit alcohol. Mixing alcohol and many drugs is also problematic. Interactions vary from inconsequential to devastating. So before you take *any* prescription or over-the-counter (OTC) drug, be sure to discuss the use of alcohol with your pharmacist and health care provider.

Cherries and cherry juice: Red cherries such as the Montmorency and Balaton contain phytochemicals called *anthocyanins.* Researchers from Michigan State University found that the antioxidant activity of the anthocyanins in cherries rivals that of vitamin E. They also inhibit the function of cyclooxygenase-2 (COX-2), an enzyme that's a major player in inflammation. The use of cherries and cherry juice is also being explored for chronic pain and inflammation such as in osteoarthritis because of this connection.

Plant stanol/sterol products such as Take Control Light and Benecol Light spreads or Minute Maid Heart Wise juice. Plant stanols and sterols are found naturally in corn, rice, soybeans, squash, other plants, and vegetable oils. They are chemically related to cholesterol yet very different in that humans absorb them poorly. Eating spread or drinking juice made with sterols or stanols blocks the absorption of both dietary and body-manufactured cholesterol from the intestine into the bloodstream, resulting in a reduction of your total and LDL blood cholesterol. Use these stanols/sterols spreads just like regular butter or margarine, on everything from toast, bagels, and oatmeal to corn on the cob, baked sweet potatoes, and steamed veggies. We recommend the light version of these spreads for their lower calories. There are no reported side effects, and studies have shown that a continuous intake of one to two servings per day can lower total cholesterol by about 10 percent (decreasing without negatively affecting HDL). If you discontinue these products, your total and LDL cholesterol may return to their previous levels. Both products can be used with statin medications.

> Look for Take Control Light and Benecol Light spreads in your grocery with margarines.

Garlic: For years garlic has been touted for its role in lowering cholesterol. A meta-analysis (review of clinical trials) published in the *Annals of Internal Medicine* found the cholesterol-lowering benefits of garlic to be only 4 to 6 percent versus the 17 to 30 percent previously thought. Alone, this benefit isn't significant, but combined with other Focus Foods such as soy, stanol/sterol spreads, and oats, the combined effects become much stronger.

One to two raw or cooked garlic cloves per day is the amount needed to derive the health benefits. Allicin, the active factor in garlic, is released and available after the clove is crushed or chewed. Yes, you may have garlic breath and even garlic body odor, so keep the breath mints and toothbrush handy. But remember that roasted garlic or garlic used in cooking is usually less offensive. More than five cloves may possibly give you gas, an upset stomach, or heartburn. Large amounts (five or more cloves) may act as a blood thinner, so if you take blood-thinning drugs such as warfarin or even aspirin or high doses of vitamin E, forget about eating large amounts of garlic. See the "Supplement" section later in the chapter, if you choose to take garlic supplements.

Soy: Soy protein (not to be confused with soy isoflavones, which are a plant estrogen) can lower cholesterol levels. Consuming soy foods four times a day (for a total of 25 grams of soy protein) tends to lower the cholesterol level about ten points in the average person. It lowers the LDL cholesterol level by 4 to 6 percent in people with very high LDL levels (160 or more).

Soy foods must contain at least 6.25 grams of soy protein per serving, and the label must state that you need to consume 25 grams of soy protein per day as part of a diet low in saturated fat, before the Food and Drug Administration (FDA) will allow a cholesterol-lowering claim on a label.

For very elevated cholesterol and LDL levels, a commitment of four servings per day is worth consideration. For others, the best use of soy is as part of the overall food portfolio. Since soy foods contain very little if any saturated fat, replacing animal protein with soy foods and incorporating soy foods such as soy milk, edamame, tofu, and soy burgers, into the diet every day helps lower the total saturated fat intake and often reduces calorie intake.

Tomatoes: Products including tomato paste, juice, sauce, and salsa contain the potent antioxidant *lycopene,* which gives these items their naturally red color. And heat-processed tomato products, such as your favorite tomato sauce, can actually contain up to six times as much lycopene as fresh tomatoes. The heat factor releases the lycopene from the tomato cell walls, making it easier to absorb in our digestive systems. Being fat soluble, lycopene is best used by the body when accompanied by a bit of healthy fat such as olive oil. A study reported in *The Journal of Nutrition* found that lycopene from tomato product consumption prevented oxidation of lipoproteins by free radicals that can result in arterial plaque formation. Lycopene is also found in watermelon, guava, and pink grapefruit.

Nuts and seeds: The negative reputation of high-fat, high-calorie nuts has been redeemed, because 1 to 2 ounces per day have been shown to lower cholesterol by 5 to 15 percent. The improvement in cholesterol results from a synergistic effect among the various powerful ingredients, including fiber, magnesium, folate, protein, monounsaturated fat, and vitamin E. The latest studies credit the "gamma" form of vitamin E in nuts, seeds, and oils, not the "alpha" form found in most vitamin E supplements, for working with other nutrients to lower cholesterol.

We're talking not just peanuts but almonds, walnuts, macadamias, and soy nuts as well. However, this is one item that demands close attention when it comes to portion size. Sesame seeds and pumpkin seeds are also great in the portions recommended in the Food List later in this chapter (see page 122). Nuts and nut butters such as peanut and cashew butter are very healthy, but to include them regularly, something else has to go, because an ounce of nuts is 160 to 180 calories. You'll notice that your NO-TIME and MORE-TIME Menus use them frequently but somewhat sparingly, such as tossed in a salad, mixed with yogurt, or on top of hot cereal.

Beans and legumes, oats, apples and other produce: Not just good fiber sources, apples, beans and legumes, oatmeal, and other fruits help to lower blood cholesterol and assist in normalizing blood glucose and insulin levels. These high-fiber foods delay stomach emptying and prevent glucose fluctuations, providing you with a feeling of satiety. Typically, high-fiber foods are lower in fat and sugar calories but rich in vitamins, minerals, antioxidants, and phytochemicals. They are also good sources of folate and vitamin B6. All of these features fit perfectly into this weight loss plan.

Currently, however, the average American eats only enough high-fiber foods to reach about 12 to 18 grams per day, a far cry from the suggested 25 to 38 grams. No wonder we are often referred to as the most constipated society!

Researchers at Tulane University who studied 10,000 men and women over twenty years found that those with the highest intake (300 mcg) of dietary folate had a 13 percent lower risk for heart disease and a 20 percent lower risk of stroke. Folate (or folic acid in supplements) brings down the homocysteine level (an amino acid that harms artery walls) in the blood. In addition to being good fiber sources, oranges, dried beans, grain products, and leafy greens are all good sources of folate. Please see Appendix F for a list of high-fiber foods.

Olive oil, olives, canola oil: These are great sources of monounsaturated fat and are rich in oleic acid, which has anti-inflammatory actions similar to those of omega-3 oils in fish. When substituted for saturated fat or polyunsaturated fat, monounsaturated fat from olives, olive oil, or canola oil has been shown to lower total cholesterol and lower LDL cholesterol without negatively affecting HDL cholesterol.

What's the big deal about substituting monounsaturated fats for saturated fats and trans fats? See Appendix E.

Seafood: The omega-3 fatty acids found in fish help protect the heart by decreasing inflammation levels in the arteries (as evidenced in lower C-reactive protein [CRP] indexes), promoting blood vessel elasticity, reducing the formation of blood clots, keeping heart rhythms stable, and lowering blood triglyceride levels.

The typical American diet is full of processed foods, which many times include corn, sunflower, and safflower oils, all high in omega-6 polyunsaturated fat. All are thought to be "heart healthy" since they don't increase blood cholesterol. Nevertheless, people should not overlook the importance of keeping the ratio of omega-6s to omega-3s within a healthy range. When omega-6s overshadow the omega-3s, COX-2 levels go up and inflammation increases. In the United States, unfortunately, the omega-6 intake is estimated to be fifteen to twenty times higher than the omega-3 intake. You can achieve a better balance and less inflammation by adding more fish and other omega-3-containing foods (such as canola oil, soybeans, walnuts, soybean oil, and flaxseed meal) to the diet while cutting back some on products including omega-6 oils.

FOCUS FOOD FREQUENCY

FOOD ITEM	FREQUENCY
Anti-inflammatory fruits/vegetables/herbs/spices	Daily
Tea: black, oolong, and green	2–3 cups per day
Purple and red grapes and grape juice	1 cup grapes or ½ cup juice 3–4 times per week
Red wine (optional)	5–6 ounces 3–4 times per week
Red cherries, cherry juice	1 cup red cherries, ¼ cup dried cherries, or ½ cup juice 3–4 times per week
Benecol Light or Take Control Light or Minute Maid Heart Wise juice	1 tablespooon 1–2 times per day 8 ounces per day
Garlic	1–2 raw or cooked cloves per day
Soy foods	At least 1 per day; 4 per day to equal 25 grams of soy protein for cholesterol-lowering effects
Tomato products	3–5 times per week
Nuts and seeds	¼ cup 3–4 times per week
Beans, oats, apples, etc.	Daily
Soybean oil, canola oil	Daily as an oil source in salad dressings or in cooking
Seafood	2–3 times per week

Begin with the Phenotype C *FAST TRACK* Two Weeks

With its quick results, the *FAST TRACK* Two Weeks gets you motivated to keep going. The *FAST TRACK* is too severe for achieving long-term changes to your phenotype, but it will jump-start your weight loss. You'll begin to feel leaner, healthier, and sexier within days. It uses the same format as the Phenotype C Diets for men and women below, with the following exceptions:

1. Omit the number of proteins, carbohydrates and fats from the Phenotype C Diet, as **boldfaced** in parentheses in the Meals and Snacks below.
2. Omit the two fist-size 👊 👊 portions of "Sweets, Treats, and Alcohol" (see page 124) allowed each week.
3. Take a multivitamin/mineral supplement as well as the recommended additional vitamin C and vitamin E daily (see "Supplements" on page 132).
4. Start Week 3 with the full Phenotype C Diet.

THE PHENOTYPE C DIET FOR WOMEN

Select your foods for each meal and snack from the Food List on page 122. Sample Menus using foods that fit the diet are on page 125.

Meal 1
1 Protein (any fist, ½ fist, or thumb[s] selection)
2 Carbohydrates
1 Fat **(omit 1 fat for *FAST TRACK* Two Weeks)**
Freebie beverages

Meal 2
2 Proteins (1 palm **or** any 2: fist, ½ fist, or thumb[s] selections) **(omit 1 protein for *FAST TRACK* Two Weeks)**
2 Carbohydrates
Freebie vegetables
1 Fat
Freebie beverages

Meal 3
2 Proteins (any 2: fist, ½ fist, or thumb[s] selections)
4 Carbohydrates **(omit 1 carbohydrate for *FAST TRACK* Two Weeks)**
Freebie vegetables
2 Fats **(omit 1 fat for *FAST TRACK* Two Weeks)**
Freebie beverages

Snack
1 Carbohydrate
Freebie beverages

THE PHENOTYPE C DIET FOR MEN

**Select your foods for each meal and snack from the Food
List on page 122. Sample menus using foods that fit the diet
are on page 128.**

Meal 1
1 Protein (any fist, ½ fist, or thumb[s] selection)
3 Carbohydrates **(omit 1 carbohydrate for *FAST TRACK* Two
  Weeks)**
1 Fat
Freebie beverages

Meal 2
2 Proteins (1 palm **or** any 2: fist, ½ fist, or thumb[s] selections)
  (omit 1 protein for *FAST TRACK* Two Weeks)
3 Carbohydrates
Freebie vegetables
2 Fats
Freebie beverages

Meal 3
2 Proteins (any 2: fist, ½ fist, or thumb[s] selections)
4 Carbohydrates **(omit 1 carbohydrate for *FAST TRACK* Two
  Weeks)**
Freebie vegetables
2 Fats **(omit 1 fat for *FAST TRACK* Two Weeks)**
Freebie beverages

Snack 1
1 Protein (any fist, ½ fist, or thumb[s] selection)
1 Carbohydrate
Freebie beverages

**Stopped losing weight? Refer to "How to Deal with Plateaus"
on page 28 and reboot your diet with another *FAST TRACK* Two
Weeks.**

FOOD LIST

Focus Foods are in **bold type.**

How much of each food should you eat? Use your hand as your guide. Eat the amount that you see; that is, the size of your fist, your palm, or your thumb.

 PALM

 FIST

 THUMB

Protein Sources

 Seafood. Poultry without skin, or lean cuts of meat such as loin, round, or cutlets of beef, pork, ham, veal, venison, lamb, etc.; cook by steaming, sautéing, broiling, or grilling. Meat alternative (**tofu, tempeh,** or other **soy** product)

 Skim milk, buttermilk, evaporated skim milk, low-fat yogurt, low-fat cottage cheese, or calcium fortified soy milk, **eggs such as Eggland's Best Eggs that are rich in omega-3 fatty acids (100 mg per egg),** ricotta cheese (fat free)

½ **Edamame, garbanzo, pinto, kidney, black, lima, or white beans; split, black-eyed, or field peas; lentils**

  Parmigiano-Reggiano, grana padana, string cheese, Neufchâtel (reduced-fat cream cheese), **soy cheese, peanut butter, almond butter or other nut butters, walnuts, almonds, Brazil nuts, cashews, chestnuts, hazelnuts, macadamia nuts, mixed nuts, peanuts, pecans, pine nuts, pistachios, soy nuts, pumpkin seeds, sunflower seeds**

 Swiss, Cheddar, mozzarella, Romano, colby, goat, Monterey Jack, feta, or Gorgonzola

Carbohydrate Sources

🐟 **Whole grain bread, corn tortilla, whole wheat tortilla, whole grain English muffin, bagel, whole wheat pita or ½ round whole grain lavash, whole grain crackers,** polenta, focaccia bread, **corn bread, whole grain muffins, whole grain waffles or pancakes**

✊ ✊ ✊ **Popped popcorn**

✊ **High-fiber cereal, muesli**

✊ **Apple, banana, berries, carambola (star fruit), cherries, citrus, grapes, kiwi fruit, melon, mango, nectarine, peach, pear, pineapple, plum**

✊ **100% fruit juice, plain, calcium-fortified, or stanol/sterol-fortified (limit to once a day)**

½ ✊ **Grits; oatmeal; Wheatena; couscous; whole wheat pasta, pasta with at least 2 grams of fiber per serving; brown rice or other whole grain; garbanzo, pinto, kidney, black, lima, or white beans; split, black-eyed, or field peas; lentils; edamame; corn; green peas; potatoes with skin; acorn or butternut squash; sweet potatoes or yams; plantain**

> Check out the *Freebie* list for lots of veggies, including salad greens, tomatoes, carrots, etc., that you don't have to limit.

✊ ✊ **Dried fruit such as raisins, cherries, blueberries, apricots, plums, figs, etc.**

✊ **Flaxseed meal, wheat germ**

Fat Sources

MONOUNSATURATED FATS

✊ ✊ **Avocado, olives, hummus, almonds, Brazil nuts, cashews, chestnuts, hazelnuts, macadamia nuts, mixed nuts, peanuts, pecans, pine nuts, pistachios, soy nuts, walnuts, pumpkin seeds, safflower seeds, sesame seeds, sunflower seeds**

✊ **Olive oil, canola oil, peanut oil, tahini paste, low–trans fat margarines such as Olivio**

Polyunsaturated Fats

👍 👍 **Benecol Light or Take Control Light spread,** salad dressing, light margarine, light mayonnaise, light salad dressing, low–trans fat margarines such as Smart Balance

👍 Benecol or Take Control spread, corn oil, safflower oil, soybean oil, sesame oil, sunflower oil, tartar sauce, salad dressing

Freebies

Beverages: Coffee, tea, or diet soft drinks up to caffeine limit of 450 mg/day, club soda, carbonated or mineral water

Veggies: Artichoke, artichoke hearts, arugula, asparagus, bean sprouts, beets, Bibb lettuce, broccoli, Brussels sprouts, carrots, cauliflower, cabbage, celery, collard greens, cucumber, endive, eggplant, escarole, green beans, green onions or scallions, green, red, or yellow pepper, kale, kohlrabi, leeks, lettuce, mixed greens, mesclun, mushrooms, mustard greens, okra, onions, pea pods, radishes, romaine, spinach, summer squash, tomato, turnips, turnip greens, water chestnuts, zucchini

Miscellaneous: Broth or bouillon, ketchup, horseradish, lemon juice, lime juice, mustard, pickles, soy sauce, taco sauce, **salsa,** vinegars, garlic, **fresh or dried herbs,** pimento, spices, **red wine used in cooking,** Worcestershire sauce, sugar substitute

Sweets, Treats, and Alcohol

The Phenotype C Diet gives you two fists ✊ ✊ of your choice per week to use as you desire. These treats are already calculated into your diet.

Whether it's a new Italian cheese, an exquisite red wine, a family birthday party or the tempting restaurant that opened down the street, the two fist-size portions of treats weekly keep you in the real world of eating and enjoying food. You may use your two fist-size portions of treats all at once, such as on a couple of glasses of a great Rosemount Shiraz. You could just as easily indulge your

> To use the two fists ✊ ✊ as treats, you don't have to subtract anything from the Phenotype C Diet.

passion with two fists worth of good chocolate eaten over the course of a week. That's the beauty of it—it's your choice.

Chocolate has flavonoids, which aid heart health by improving blood vessel function, specifically blood vessel dilation or elasticity. And although chocolate is high in fat, about one third of the fat is stearic acid, which doesn't cause an increase in your blood cholesterol. Cocoa powder and chocolate also add trace minerals to the diet, such as magnesium, copper, and potassium. Currently, Dove Dark Chocolates contain a flavonol-rich chocolate called Cocoapro that is being investigated in a number of studies.

Don't forget, alcohol can wreak havoc on your blood triglyceride level. So if you tend to have high triglycerides, consider limiting or even omitting alcohol. Alcohol's love-hate relationship with many drugs can also be a big issue. Interactions can vary from inconsequential to devastating, so if you take *any* prescription or over-the-counter (OTC) drugs, be sure to discuss the use of alcohol with your pharmacist and health care provider.

SAMPLE MENUS

On days when you're rushed, use the NO-TIME Menus. MORE-TIME Menus are for days when you can cook leisurely. The menus are also meant to serve as a guide for eating out.

NO-TIME Menu C for Women

MEAL 1

Lemon yogurt (low-fat, low-sugar or sugar free; eat before you leave or at work)

Quaker Cinnamon Oat Squares (put into a Baggie for munching on the way to work)

Banana (eat before you leave or at work)

Freebie beverages

or

Creamsicle smoothie (If you love smoothies, here's how to substitute fruit for the cereal. See NO-TIME recipes in Appendix C for more smoothie ideas.)

You can buy flaxseed already ground in many groceries and health food stores, or you can grind your own flaxseed in your coffee grinder. If it is ground, the body utilizes the ALA, lignans, and other healthy components, but if it is not ground, the flaxseed passes through the body as a fiber source only.

 Vanilla yogurt (low-fat; can use frozen yogurt and no ice)

½ Orange juice

Banana

Flaxseed meal or wheat germ

Combine all ingredients in a blender. Add crushed ice or cubes and blend for 30–45 seconds. Pour into cup and go.

or

Go to a smoothie bar and choose a *small* one with similar ingredients.

Commercial smoothies are typically packed with calories, so order the small size. Forgo the add-ons, such as protein powder, herbs, and other supplements. Try to match your ingredients with those of your diet plan.

MEAL 2

Spicy black bean soyburger (such as Morningstar) with:

Sunflower seed bread

Freebie Fresh tomato, lettuce, and onion slices

Freebie Salsa

Freebie Hot mustard

Freebie Baby carrots, julienne red or green peppers, and cauliflower florets with:

Ranch dressing (light)

Freebie beverages

Meal 3

 Maple-Ginger Salmon (see NO-TIME Recipes, in Appendix C)

 Cinnamon acorn squash (microwave quick fix):

Freebie Red or green leaf lettuce with:

> *Freebie* Water chestnuts, sliced cucumber, and chopped celery

Slice squash in half. Remove seeds and membranes. Place cut side down in a microwave-safe dish. Cook on high for about 8 minutes. Time may vary with ovens. While warm, add 1 teaspoon Take Control Light or Benecol Light spread. Sprinkle with cinnamon as desired.

> Balsamic-Dill Vinaigrette (see NO-TIME recipes in Appendix C, page 258) or balsamic vinaigrette such as Newman's Own

 Fruit and bran muffin (can use a quick mix or buy a bakery muffin)

Freebie beverages

To save time, use a quick muffin mix such as Sun-Maid Honey Raisin Bran, which is lower in hydrogenated fat than other mixes. Add ³⁄₄–1 cup dried fruit such as raisins, dates, or apricots to the mix prior to baking, and be sure to use preferred oil. If you buy a bran muffin from a store or bakery, check the ingredients label for the fat source or ask.

Snack

 Gala or Golden Delicious apple

 Almond butter (peanut or cashew butter is fine too)

Freebie beverages

MORE-TIME Menu C for Women

Meal 1

 Soy sausage links (such as Morningstar)

 Buckwheat pancakes with:

> Fresh blueberries

> Take Control Light or Benecol Light

Hot green, black, or oolong tea or other *Freebie* beverages

Cook several pancakes on the griddle and warm for breakfast on other days. To save time, look for buckwheat pancake mix such as Arrowhead Mills or Hodgson Mill.

MEAL 2

Freebie Spring mix salad with:

 Grilled fresh tuna

> Try some of the flavored oils such as Olio Santo blood orange olive oil or lemon olive oil from Williams-Sonoma stores.

Freebie vegetables

 Blood orange–infused olive oil

Freebie Balsamic vinegar

 Warm pumpernickel-rye bread with Take Control Light or Benecol Light spread

Freebie beverages

MEAL 3

 Lime-grilled boneless chicken breast/tenderloins with:

  Avocado served on brown rice (use the quick-cook microwave rice)

 Roasted Sicilian Vegetables (see MORE-TIME Recipes in Appendix C)

Freebie beverages

SNACK

 Dried cherries **or** purple grape juice **or** red wine

Freebie beverages

NO-TIME MENU C FOR MEN

MEAL 1

 Lemon yogurt (low-fat, low-sugar, or sugar free; eat before you leave or at work)

Quaker Cinnamon Oat Squares **and** 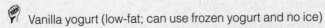 dried fruit such as raisins, cherries, or apricots (put in a Baggie to munch on the way to work)

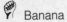 Banana (eat before you leave or at work)

Freebie beverages

or

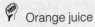 Creamsicle smoothie: (If you love smoothies, here's how to substitute fruit for the cereal. See NO-TIME Recipes, in Appendix C, for more smoothie ideas.)

> Vanilla yogurt (low-fat; can use frozen yogurt and no ice)
>
> Orange juice
>
> Banana
>
> Flaxseed meal or wheat germ

Combine all ingredients in a blender. Add crushed ice or cubes and blend for 30–45 seconds. Pour into cup and go.

You can buy flaxseed already ground in many groceries and health food stores, or you can grind your own flaxseed in your coffee grinder. If it is ground, the body utilizes the ALA, lignans, and other healthy components, but if it is not ground, the flaxseed passes through the body as a fiber source only.

or

Go to a smoothie bar and choose a small one with similar ingredients.

Commercial smoothies are typically packed with calories, so order the small size. Forgo the add-ons, such as protein powder, herbs, and other supplements. Try to match your ingredients with those of your diet plan.

MEAL 2

 Spicy black bean soyburger (such as Morningstar) with:

>   Sunflower seed bread

> Deli Swiss cheese, thin slice

> *Freebie* Fresh tomato, lettuce, and onion slices

> *Freebie* Salsa

> *Freebie* Hot mustard

Freebie Red or green leaf lettuce with:

> *Freebie* Baby carrots, julienne red or green peppers, or cauliflower florets with:

>   Ranch dressing (light)

 Nectarine

Freebie beverages

MEAL 3

 Maple-Ginger Salmon (see NO-TIME recipes in Appendix C)

 Cinnamon acorn squash (microwave quick fix)

Freebie Broccoli florets (use frozen broccoli; add minced fresh garlic and a spritz of olive oil and microwave 3–5 minutes on high; sprinkle with peanuts)

 Tropical fruit salad (pick up precut fruit at grocery such as purple or red seedless grapes, pineapple, kiwi, mango, watermelon)

Slice squash in half. Remove seeds and membranes. Place cut side down in a microwave-safe dish. Cook on high for about 8 minutes. Time may vary with ovens. While warm, add 1 teaspoon Take Control Light or Benecol Light spread. Sprinkle with cinnamon as desired.

Fruit and bran muffin (can use a quick mix or buy a bakery muffin)

SNACK

 Gala or Golden Delicious apple

 Almond butter (peanut or cashew butter is fine too)

Freebie beverages

MORE-TIME Menu C for Men

MEAL 1

 Soy sausage links (such as Morningstar)

  Buckwheat pancakes with:

      Fresh blueberries

      Take Control Light or Benecol Light

> Cook several pancakes on the griddle and warm for breakfast on other days. To save time, look for buckwheat pancake mix such as Arrowhead Mills or Hodgson Mill.

Hot green, black, or oolong tea or other *Freebie* beverages

MEAL 2

Freebie Spring mix salad with:

      Grilled fresh tuna

      Mandarin oranges

      Sesame seeds (toast for intense flavor)

> To save time, use a quick muffin mix such as Sun-Maid Honey Raisin Bran, which is lower in hydrogenated fat than other mixes. Add ¾–1 cup dried fruit such as raisins, dates, or apricots to the mix prior to baking, and be sure to use preferred oil. If you buy a bran muffin from the store or bakery, check the ingredients label for the fat source or ask.

Freebie vegetables

 Lemon-infused olive oil

Freebie Balsamic vinegar

 Warm pumpernickel-rye bread with Take Control Light or Benecol Light spread

Freebie beverages

Try some of the flavored oils such as Olio Santo blood orange olive oil or lemon olive oil from Williams-Sonoma stores.

MEAL 3

 Lime-grilled boneless chicken breast/tenderloins with:

 Avocado served on brown rice (use quick-cook microwave brown rice; for more flavor substitute orange juice for the water)

Roasted Sicilian Vegetables (see MORE-TIME Recipes in Appendix C)

Fresh raspberries with Chambord (optional)

Freebie beverages

SNACK

Barbecue soy nuts (such as GeniSoy) **or** pecans

Dried cherries **or** purple grape juice **or** red wine

Freebie beverages

Supplements

Benecol Soft Chews: Benecol is a dietary supplement that contains plant stanol esters, just like the spread discussed in the Focus Foods section. If you're using a statin medication to lower your cholesterol, Benecol supplements can produce additional cholesterol-lowering benefits since they work to block cholesterol absorption, and the statins work by decreasing cholesterol production. However, it is recommended that you use either the spread or the supplement, *not* both.

Omega-3 fatty acids: These are fats such as eicosapentaenoic acid (EPA) and docosahexaeoic acid (DHA), which are common in the oils of fish. If you do not eat fish, consider taking a fish oil supplement. Taking supplements containing omega-3 fatty acids, up to 1 gram per day, has been shown to reduce blood triglyceride levels, raise HDL levels, "thin" the blood, reduce homocysteine levels, and have anti-inflammatory effects, which lowers the risk of atherosclerosis.

Choose a supplement that, taken three times a day, provides a **total** of approximately 900 mg per day of EPA and DHA. Most 1,000 mg capsules contain 180 mg EPA and 120 mg DHA each. At these recommended doses, side effects such as fishy aftertaste, stomach distress, or a rise in LDL cholesterol are minimal. As doses increase above these recommended levels, the side effects increase. *If you are taking prescription blood thinners such as warfarin (Coumadin) or heparin or are expecting to undergo surgery, ask your physician before taking fish oil supplements.*

Niacin: As early as the 1950s, niacin at high doses (1–3 g) was found to lower blood cholesterol. Since the recommended dietary intake as a vitamin is only 14–16 mg per day, in such large amounts, niacin works as a drug, also lowering triglycerides and LDL cholesterol and boosting HDL cholesterol, something most statin drugs don't do, except for atorvastatin (Lipitor). This makes niacin one of the few drugs that improves all four lipid components.

But because niacin does not reduce LDL cholesterol as much as the statins and LDL is the best-known risk predictor today, niacin is not considered to be an initial treatment. The statin drugs such as Lipitor, Mevacor, Lescol, Pravachol, and Zocor are the drugs of choice for lowering high LDL cholesterol when diet and lifestyle changes haven't reduced it to recommended levels. These drugs act by inhibiting the liver enzyme called HMG CoA reductase, which is responsible for producing cholesterol. They also stabilize deposits on artery walls, thus preventing clot formation, promote the growth of new vessels, relax blood vessels, and reduce inflammation. Grapefruit juice should not be consumed when taking statin medications.

Niacin is sometimes used in combination with statin drugs when triglycerides are above 250 mg/dl. The extended-release form usually prevents the common side effects of flushing and potential liver problems. If you are taking niacin at such high doses, your physician should monitor liver enzymes routinely.

MAJOR RISK FACTORS THAT AFFECT LDL CHOLESTEROL GOALS

Age: Men ≥ 45 years, Women ≥ 55 years
Cigarette smoking
High blood pressure (BP >140/90)
HDL cholesterol below 40 mg/dl
Family history of premature heart disease:
    < Age 55 in father or brother
    < Age 65 in mother or sister
The latest National Cholesterol Education Program Expert Panel report recommends considering drug treatment in people with:
    Heart disease or diabetes
    Three or more of the above risks when their LDL cholesterol
       is ≥ 130 mg/dl,
    Two or more of these risks when their LDL cholesterol is
       ≥ 160 mg/dl
    None or one of these risks when their LDL cholesterol is
       ≥ 190 mg/dl

Garlic: Garlic supplements require the enzyme alliinase to convert alliin to allicin once the pill is swallowed and touches liquid. The problem with supplements is that the alliinase enzyme is destroyed by stomach acid, so the true availability of allicin is hard to quantify. A study in the *Journal of the American College of Nutrition* reported that *enteric-coated* garlic supplements reduced total cholesterol and LDL by 4 to 6 percent. Some garlic pills such as Kwai are enteric-coated to bypass the stomach acid and remain intact until they get to the intestine. The garlic odor is mostly eliminated, and the minimal therapeutic benefits are protected.

However, the more we learn about medical nutrition therapy, the more we realize that there are many compounds in food, beyond the ones currently known, which may be active in the body. For example, a garlic supplement called Kyolic Extract utilizes the ingredient S-allyl-cysteine (SAC) instead of allicin.

If you are also taking aspirin, vitamin E, or other blood-thinning medication, ask your physician before beginning garlic supplements, since they also affect clotting time. Adding garlic to your diet as a focus food is a better choice in this scenario.

Psyllium (such as Metamucil): Two to 10 grams of psyllium a day have been shown to reduce total and LDL cholesterol up to 10 percent. Psyllium has been used as a high-fiber treatment for constipation in the United States for many years. It's sold over the counter as a laxative in powder or in wafer form and as an ingredient in the breakfast cereal Bran Buds. As with any fiber source, whether food or supplement, you must drink more water when taking it and add the fiber to your diet gradually.

SUPPLEMENT RECOMMENDATIONS AND DOSES

SUPPLEMENT	DOSE
Multivitamin/mineral	Daily
Vitamin C	250 mg daily
Vitamin E:	200 IU mixed tocopherols for women daily; 400 IU mixed tocopherols for men daily
Benacol Soft Chews	1–2 Soft Chews per day with meals or snacks if not using Benecol Light or Take Control Light spread or Minute Maid Heart Wise juice
Omega-3 or fish oil supplements	The latest American Heart Association recommendations are: 2–4 grams of supplemental fish oil daily if you have blood triglycerides above 200 mg/dl 1 gram (1,000 mg) of EPA and DHA fish oil daily if you have heart disease; to get this amount, take a 1,000 mg fish oil capsule three times per day with meals, since most 1,000 mg capsules contain only 180 mg EPA and 120 mg DHA each

(continued on next page)

SUPPLEMENT	**DOSE**
Niacin	1–4 grams daily of niacin, niacinamide, or inositol hexaniacinate for elevated triglycerides; your liver enzymes should be monitored by your physician
Enteric-coated garlic	900 mg daily of a tablet that contains 1.3% alliin, the sulfur-containing substance of which allicin is a breakdown product
Psyllium	1 round teaspoon (3–4 grams) taken 1–3 times a day; start at the lowest dose and increase your water intake by 8 oz for each teaspoon used; or take 2–4 wafers providing 3 grams each

The Phenotype C Maintenance Diet

Remember when you started on the Phenotype C Diet? In a few days, something inside just seemed to click and you began to lose weight, feel better, and feel healthier. That will not change. When you reach your weight goal, you are ready to move on to the Phenotype C Maintenance Diet. The diet has the same backbone Focus Foods. Still tailored to your genetic blueprint, it will keep you satisfied and your weight constant. A high level of physical activity or exercise is the single best predictor of keeping lost weight off. So keep moving!

THE PHENOTYPE C
MAINTENANCE DIET FOR WOMEN

Meal 1
1 Protein (any fist, ½ fist, or thumb[s] selection)
3 Carbohydrates
2 Fats
Freebie beverages

Meal 2
2 Proteins (1 palm **or** any 2: fist, ½ fist, or thumb[s] selections)
2 Carbohydrates
Freebie vegetables
1 Fat
Freebie beverages

Meal 3
2 Proteins (any 2: fist, ½ fist, or thumb[s] selections)
4 Carbohydrates
Freebie vegetables
4 Fats
Freebie beverages

Snack
2 Carbohydrates
Freebie beverages

THE PHENOTYPE C
MAINTENANCE DIET FOR MEN

Meal 1
1 Protein (any fist, ½ fist, or thumb[s] selection)
3 Carbohydrates
1 Fat
Freebie beverages

Meal 2
2 Proteins (1 palm **or** any 2: fist, ½ fist, or thumb[s] selections)
4 Carbohydrates
Freebie vegetables
3 Fats
Freebie beverages

Meal 3
2 Proteins (any 2: fist, ½ fist, or thumb[s] selections)
5 Carbohydrates
Freebie vegetables
3 Fats
Freebie beverages

Snack 1
1 Protein (any fist, ½ fist, or thumb[s] selection)
1 Carbohydrate
Freebie beverages

CHAPTER 7

The Phenotype D Diet

OUTSMARTING DIABETES-LINKED
WEIGHT GAIN

Tina Marie's Story

"When those test results came back, I began to panic. My mind immediately went to my mom, and I thought to myself—I'm becoming her!"

Tina Marie is a Phenotype D. Her mother, to whom she was very close, struggled with vision problems as well as numbness in her fingers and toes, then was diagnosed with type 2 diabetes after age 50. When Tina Marie went for a physical right after her fiftieth birthday, she found out that her blood triglycerides and glucose were elevated. She was also about 40 pounds overweight—as Tina Marie put it, "Twenty pounds for each of my children."

Her glucose level was not yet high enough for a diabetes diagnosis, but Tina Marie knew it was a wake-up call. She was not surprised when we talked about her mom and the risks Tina Marie now faced. "I absolutely love carbs, and when you look at what I wrote down in my Food Record, you'll see that I ate lots of pasta, bread, potatoes, corn, and rice. My husband and I are also very worried about our son right now. He is in the Special Forces and overseas. We don't know where he is or if he's okay. The more I worry, the more I reach for the carbs. I know this is affecting both my weight and my blood sugar. I need to be there for my son, and I don't want to end up like my mom—what do I do?"

If you are overweight and a Phenotype D, you answered "yes" to some of these statements in the Phenotype Assessment:

- My mother has or had diabetes or metabolic syndrome.
- My fasting blood sugar is or has been **too high,** above 100 mg/dl.
- My blood triglycerides have been **above** 150 mg/dl.
- I am taking a blood sugar–lowering medication or using insulin.
- I would describe my exercise level as inactive.

STEP ONE: UNDERSTANDING YOUR PHENOTYPE

Phenotype Ds gain weight in connection with a genetic tendency for elevated blood glucose levels and diabetes. If you have higher-than-normal blood glucose levels, you or your mother has been diagnosed with type 2 diabetes, and you carry too many pounds around your middle, this is your phenotype. Diabetes, and even metabolic syndrome and prediabetes, may increase your vulnerability to numerous other diseases. Research has established that diabetes is now the most common health problem tied to weight gain, comprising an interdependent genetic grouping we call Phenotype D.

Diabetes Can Starve Your Cells

To grasp diabetes' relationship to weight gain, one must begin with *glucose* and *insulin.* Our digestive systems break all foods down into glucose, a simple sugar in the blood known as "blood glucose" or "blood sugar." Insulin is the hormone responsible for ushering this glucose through the bloodstream and into our cells to be used as energy. In people with diabetes, this mechanism is impaired.

For our clients and patients, we use a "lock-and-key" analogy to explain the way insulin works. Hormones such as insulin are like passkeys, purposely formed to unlock only specific locks. The "locks" are *receptors* on cell surfaces, each available to be unlocked by certain hormones. To the correct passkeys, these locklike receptors remain available as an avenue of entry into the cells—as long as the cells stay healthy and the receptors viable. As a passkey, insulin's role is to unlock fat cells, muscle cells, and other cells. When insulin attaches to the insulin receptor on these cell surfaces, it triggers chemical reactions inside that allow glucose to enter and provide those cells with energy.

Type 2 diabetes originates with one of two problems: either the pancreas, where insulin is produced, does not produce enough insulin to meet the cells' demands, or cell-surface insulin receptors are hampered in their ability to recognize the insulin passkey. They reject glucose, because the passkey doesn't fit.

This latter condition is called "insulin resistance." If you as a Phenotype D are insulin-resistant, your cells respond poorly to the action of insulin. Following a meal, glucose accumulates in your bloodstream because it isn't able to get into the cells, raising your blood sugar levels, perhaps dangerously high. You thus have a higher level of glucose circulating in the blood, signaling for yet more insulin to be released from the pancreas to help shuttle the glucose into the cells.

Your Weight, Diabetes, and Food Choices

Ten to 25 percent of the adult population may be insulin-resistant to some degree. Weight gain can lead to insulin resistance and diabetes because the insulin receptors on cells no longer function when the cells increase in size. When people gain too much weight, in effect it *distorts* the insulin receptor lock's keyhole. The key no longer fits the lock. The insulin arrives, but its movement into the cell is impeded and this sends the blood glucose level soaring.

Worse, the ready availability of refined carbohydrates in snacks and junk food exacerbates the problem. Carbohydrates, particularly refined carbohydrates, are more rapidly converted to glucose than protein or fat, and in Phenotype Ds, the compromised insulin receptors are unable to clear the entry of that readily available glucose into the cells.

Phenotype Ds are also especially vulnerable to the damaging effects of free radicals, the unstable molecules that can result from stress and exposure to pollutants. Free radicals oxidize cells similarly to the way rust oxidizes metal. If cells are not protected by the protective shield supplied by adequate antioxidants (phytochemicals from fresh fruits and vegetables), their ability to function normally will be depleted by exposure to free radicals over time. Cellular oxidative damage is higher in people with diabetes because diabetes itself is a state of increased oxidative stress.

Knowing Your Blood Glucose Level

There's an obvious correlation between weight gain and diabetes. According to the American Diabetes Association, about 90 percent of people newly diagnosed with type 2 diabetes are overweight. Sixteen million may be "in the queue" with *prediabetes* (higher-than-normal blood glucose levels but not in the diagnostic category for diabetes). Prediabetics can prevent or delay the development of type 2 diabetes and cut the risk of developing it in half by following the Phenotype D Diet and losing 5 to 10 percent of their body weight.

WHAT IS OPTIMAL BLOOD GLUCOSE?

Classification	Fasting Blood Glucose
Optimal	Below 100 mg/dl
Prediabetes	100–125 mg/dl
Diabetes	Above 126 mg/dl

Your blood glucose level is the telltale indicator of your diabetes risk. This must be a *fasting blood sample*, meaning that you must not eat for 12 hours prior to the test. When your fasting blood glucose levels are above 126 mg/dl on more than one test, diabetes is diagnosed.

A major problem is that people often have elevated blood sugar for months, maybe years, without realizing it or the risks. And the risks are huge. For Phenotype Ds, elevated blood sugar puts you on a collision course with diabetes, and untreated diabetes can generate heart or kidney disease, high blood pressure, stroke, damage to the eyes and nerves, circulatory problems, and even loss of limbs. Therefore, if you are a Phenotype D and have a family history of diabetes, you should get regular blood glucose tests.

Metabolic Syndrome

Tony's Story

"Even though my mother has diabetes, I never thought it would happen to me."

"I've always been healthy, exercised regularly, but struggled to keep my weight down," Tony told us. "In my family, a meal wasn't a meal if it didn't include dessert, and I love sweets. I had six brothers and sisters, and we didn't waste food. So, I learned to clean my plate early on. I gained a lot of weight in my late twenties after getting married and having our son. But I lost it when we divorced. I made up my mind to get fit, and that's when I started running. Over the next twenty years, however, as my business grew and I became more successful, I slowly put the pounds back on. My knees gave way and I couldn't run anymore. I went from 190 to 225 pounds."

Tony often ate while working and munched into the night as he continued on the computer. His evening meal became a series of snacks such as popcorn, heated burritos from the microwave, and food he picked up on the way home. Tony wasn't aware of what or how much he was really eating, nor did this eat/work scenario leave him satisfied.

"When I finally had a physical, the doctor told me I had the classic 'metabolic syndrome.' What in the world is that? I had never heard of it, and it sounded bad. The doctor told me my triglycerides were high, my fasting blood sugars were high, and my extra weight was all right around my middle. I was well on the way to diabetes. Even though my mother has diabetes, I never thought it would happen to me."

One common signpost experienced by many Phenotype Ds whose blood sugar is elevated over a period of time is a condition called *metabolic syndrome.* It is a cluster of metabolic symptoms, including high blood glucose levels, dyslipidemia, insulin resistance, hypertension, and abdominal obesity. Untreated, metabolic syndrome can lead to diabetes, heart disease, and stroke. This was the direction Tony was headed in.

There are twice as many people who carry the genetic risk for type 2 diabetes as those who have the disease. This disparity clearly demonstrates that your eating habits and behaviors (what scientists call your "environment") can modify your risk even when the genetic factors are present. Even so, the number of people being diagnosed with diabetes is rapidly in-

WHAT ARE TRIGLYCERIDES, AND WHY ARE THEY IMPORTANT IN METABOLIC SYNDROME?

Triglycerides are the chemical form in which most fat exists in food as well as in the body. They are found in increased levels in the blood following the digestion of fats in the intestine but are also made in the body from other energy sources like carbohydrates. Calories ingested in a meal and not used immediately by the tissues are converted to triglycerides and transported to fat cells to be stored as a potential energy source in adipose tissue (fat stored in the body). Triglycerides are released from fat tissue to meet the body's needs for energy between meals. The level of triglycerides rises in Phenotype Ds with metabolic syndrome when they consume excess calories from alcohol, refined carbohydrate, and fat in a condition called *dyslipidemia.* High levels of triglycerides increase the risk of a heart attack.

WHAT ARE HDL AND LDL, AND WHAT DO THEY HAVE TO DO WITH METABOLIC SYNDROME?

HDL stands for *high-density lipoprotein,* and it is a protective cholesterol. It is the particle in the blood that removes cholesterol from the arteries and takes it to the liver, which then processes it to be removed from the body. The higher the HDL level, the better. LDL stands for *low-density lipoprotein,* and it is the carrier for cholesterol in the blood. An elevated level of LDL, the damaging cholesterol, indicates that fat is being deposited in the arteries, increasing the risk of a heart attack. *Hyperlipidemia* is low HDL combined with elevated cholesterol, LDL, and high triglycerides. People with metabolic syndrome often have hyperlipidemia and an increased risk of heart disease.

creasing, due predominantly to less healthful trends in eating and lifestyle. Our genes have not changed; our environment has.

The incidence of diabetes and metabolic syndrome has soared commensurate with affluence. The British journal *Nature* attributes the affluence link to the "thrifty gene." The thrifty gene promotes the storage of fat, thus allowing people with the gene to survive periods of famine. Unfortunately, in times of plenty, the thrifty gene is a setup for weight gain, insulin resistance, obesity, and diabetes. Not only are we affluent, but we sit still at work, at home, and in the car. Being sedentary, we risk even more weight gain.

IF YOU HAVE THREE OR MORE OF THE FOLLOWING SYMPTOMS, YOU HAVE METABOLIC SYNDROME:

Abdominal obesity (waist measurement):

Men	> 40 inches
Women	> 35 inches
Triglycerides	> 150 mg/dl
HDL cholesterol:	
Men	< 40 mg/dl
Women	< 50 mg/dl
Blood pressure	≥ 130/85
Fasting blood glucose	≥ 100 mg/dl

Because you now recognize how weight gain elevates your blood glucose and high blood glucose may lead to a host of other weight-related problems, isn't it time to minimize the impact of this "obsolete" gene and start activating your healthful genes?

STEP TWO: KEEPING A FOOD RECORD

As part of the phenotype-based program, keeping a Food Record will help you keep track of how changing your food choices, portions, and eating habits affects your health and weight. Just as the data that scientists log and analyze demonstrate the validity of their experiments, your thinking about your diet and your record of what you eat will underscore why you are succeeding as time passes. We promise you that you will quickly see positive results.

Now that you understand the scientific correlation of your diabetes risk to your weight gain, you can see how important it is to monitor your carbohydrate intake. The record-keeping process, and the learning that goes with it, will turn you into a bit of an expert about the sugar and fiber content of foods. And it will help you understand the Phenotype D Food List and follow your diet to cut carbs, lose weight, and control your blood sugar.

READING FOOD LABELS, FOR PHENOTYPE DS

Examine the label section entitled "Nutrition Facts." Look under "Total Carbohydrate" and note the grams of "Dietary Fiber" and "Sugars." "Ingredients" are listed in descending order from most to least. Aim for a minimum of 2 grams of fiber per serving, with more being better. If sugar is the first, second, or third ingredient, that food is not on your Phenotype D Food List. Save those foods for your two fists 🖐 🖐 from "Sweets, Treats, and Alcohol." Although the sugar content is listed in grams, you can convert it to teaspoons if you divide the number of grams by four. For example, if a cup of your favorite cereal has 10 grams of sugar, this is equal to 2.5 teaspoons. Caution, however: There are many sweeteners that are basically the same as sugar and should be counted as such. For example, high-fructose corn syrup is often used in soft drinks and as a sweetening ingredient in processed foods. Honey, molasses, maple syrup, corn syrup, and brown sugar are all sweeteners similar to sugar.

First, for at least two weeks, keep a list of all the breads, pastas, rice, potatoes, corn, sweets, fruits, juices, and sweetened beverages you eat or drink. Consuming more fiber and less total carbohydrates, especially non-nutrient dense sugars, is the goal. Generally, the more processed a food item is, the less fiber and potentially more sugar it contains. Therefore, you must read food labels very carefully.

Your Food Record should look like this:

CARBOHYDRATE RECORD

Carb Foods	High Fiber	Fiber Grams	Processed/Sugar	Grams
Breakfast bar		2	✓	12
Oat Squares cereal	✓	5		2.5

To find unprocessed high-fiber foods, please consult Appendix F.

In addition, make some notes to yourself about what, how much, and when you eat in your Food Record.

Barbara's Story

"I gained weight when I first went to college, the famous 'freshman 15.' I ate at the all-you-can-eat campus cafeteria most of the time and didn't pay much attention, just filled up. In my third year, my new roommate, Sally, was really into fitness and health, so I joined the gym with her and lost the extra weight over the next six months. After college, I got my first job at the bank about the same time that my new husband started his construction business. We felt like we were finally on our way. Our families lived nearby, and we would go to one or the other for dinners during the week or on Sunday.

"Suddenly, instead of walking all over campus or riding my bike, I was sitting at the computer or standing for most of the day. That's when my weight really went up. By the time I was twenty-five, I weighed almost fifty pounds more than I had weighed in college. My husband was heavier, too, but not that much heavier. I hated the way I looked and was afraid to get pregnant because I would gain even more weight. My doctor told me I was on the verge of having diabetes, and that was the last straw. I knew we had diabetes in the family, but I never thought I would get it."

Barbara decided to list the five most important things in her life. Then she made another list of all the things she was doing in the day and compared it to her priorities. Immediately, she saw that she was letting her weight get in the way of achieving one of those priorities: having a baby. She knew things had to change. Deciding to lose weight and setting a goal to become pregnant in about six months gave her the incentive she needed to make positive, deliberate changes.

STEP THREE: DEVELOPING POSITIVE NONFOOD WEIGHT LOSS TRIGGERS

Stories similar to Barbara and Tony's are replayed every day. Life goes from being less structured and full of physical activity during college to long, sedentary work hours, skipped meals during the day, no exercise, and overeating at night. Over the years of working with people in Phenotype D, however, we know from experience how effective diet and new routines can be in turning lives around. With so much evidence that people with diabetes can control their health risks with better routines or behaviors, it is clear that Phenotype Ds must implement some real changes, in addition to eating habits, if they are to regain control over their weight. The Phenotype D Diet detailed in this chapter changes the three food-related negative triggers from the Weight Trigger Quiz into positive triggers: best food choices, structured meals, and portion control. Changing your nonfood related weight gain to weight loss triggers will also be instrumental in losing weight.

Review your answers to the Weight Trigger Quiz's nonfood categories: "Stress," "No Regular Exercise," and "Increasingly Sedentary Lifestyle." Doubtless, you'll find hints for changes you could make. Barbara, for her part, answered "true" to eight out of ten indicators in the quiz's "Stress" category, because her weight gain and diabetes risk was causing her to delay starting a family and her husband was not happy about it. Our client Tony had decreased his exercise so much when he had knee surgery that he answered "true" to six out of ten indicators in the "No Regular Exercise" category, even though he still thought of himself as active.

Changing negative behaviors goes well beyond crafting good intentions. It is much easier to stay in a rut—even an unhappy rut—than to change, because change can be uncomfortable. It takes a purposeful effort on your part. This is not a matter of having or not having willpower. You must first set a goal to make "deliberate changes." Set nonfood incentives, implement one at a time only, and reward yourself as you progress. Our experience is that it typically takes three to four weeks for a single change to become a real part of your life. Therefore, it is best to focus on one change at a time and incorporate it into your daily routine until it becomes habit, before moving to the next change. The results are definitely worth the effort. One of Barbara's first deliberate changes was to meet a neighbor three days a week after work for an hour long walk. She began to look forward to the time to get outside, destress, and talk over problems from work with her friend.

Start a "wish list" of rewards to keep you motivated, and choose an item off the list every time one of your deliberate changes becomes part of your lifestyle—permanently. Do not expect to be perfect, because you may use the first time you bungle your effort as an excuse to quit. Just decide to change and continue to stay the course. Take a look at these strategies for turning off your greatest weight gain triggers.

Reduce Your Stress

Stress causes weight gain in two ways: it leads to stress eating, and surges of the stress hormone cortisol compound the weight gain. When you are stressed, the liver receives a signal to send glucose to the bloodstream so it can be used for the "fight-or-flight" response. When stress hormones such as cortisol are elevated, extra glucose (unused by the liver and muscles) characteristically ends up stored as fat around your middle.

First use your carbohydrate Food Record to identify the patterns of stress-eating wherein you may be overdoing processed carbs and high-sugar foods. Then develop positive strategies, using the following recommendations, to help you deal with stress, anxiety, and frustration more effectively. Replace stress eating with positive stress management techniques, such as taking a walk or a swim, reading a book, talking with a friend, or getting out in the yard and pulling weeds. Tina Marie, for her part, began walking to help her deal with her concerns about her son in the military. This change mitigated the stress, and the exercise turned her weight gain trigger into a weight loss trigger.

- Eat only as a conscious, planned, and deliberate event, not as something you do when you are stressed. Tony, as an example, no longer eats all day and night as he works but stops work to eat on a regular schedule.
- Wean yourself from stress eating by continuing to write down what, how much, and when you eat in your Food Record. Having to be accountable will help you change what and when you munch.
- Make Phenotype D Focus Foods your choices when stress makes you feel that you need something to eat, and use your fist portions to regulate the amounts of sweets, treats, and alcohol you consume.

- Set aside a regular worry time, scheduled at a time when you will be at your best. When Tina Marie was tempted to overeat, or lay awake at night worrying about her son, she learned to put her negative thoughts aside until her scheduled worry time first thing each morning. She found that mornings worked best for her, because she was fresh and more alert than later in the day. Others of our clients use the morning shower or evening bath and look at their worry list before they get in. They use that time to brainstorm solutions while the warm water relaxes them.
- If your stress leads to an episode of overeating, please don't give up. When Barbara first started the Phenotype D Diet, she had dinner out with friends and ate more than her palm- or fist-sized portions. She felt guilty and angry at herself and told us she had already "blown the diet." We helped her reframe her view to "I didn't make the best choices, but it is *not* a reason to give up and quit." The next day she was to go right back to the diet and go on with the plan. She left aside her regrets and guilt, because it was the best way to accomplish her weight loss goal.
- Enlist the help of your family and friends, or see if the entire family can make the change together. Change affects everyone in your family and friends closest to you. Many people will start to make a change, only to go back to their old ways if they get flack from family and friends. By asking for everyone's help, there will be no surprises and less resistance. In the long haul, support from those around you will be crucial to your success.
- Find a relaxation technique that works for you. It can be listening to music, aromatherapy, doing yoga or tai chi, deep breathing, or laughing. Make these a regular part of each day. Tina Marie began listening to music instead of the news in the car on the way to and from work. "I like the calming sounds of classical music," she said. "Listening to the news just makes me depressed and anxious."

Develop an Active Lifestyle

The more active you are, the less time you'll have to sit around and eat. You'll also be burning calories. Here are a few ideas for incorporating more movement into your daily regime:

- Turn off the television or computer at least three nights a week and plan other activities.
- If you also spend time at work sitting in front of a computer, plan regular breaks to stretch and interrupt the pattern of sitting. Set a

timer on your PDA or computer to remind you to get up and move.

- Keep a bottle of water on the desk. Tony said, "I drink because it's there to remind me I should. A side effect is that if I drink enough water, I have to get up from my desk to go to the bathroom at intervals, which is a good time to stretch—another smart thing for us desk jockeys to do."
- Carry your own groceries and other heavy items when possible, to increase your strength, build your muscle mass and increase your metabolism.

Exercise Regularly

The benefits of regular exercise are well documented for preventing and treating the metabolic changes associated with Phenotype D. Exercise improves carbohydrate metabolism and insulin sensitivity and has been shown to prevent or delay the onset of type 2 diabetes, because it lowers glucose levels. Exercise also lowers LDL cholesterol levels and increases the positive HDL cholesterol in your blood, diminishing the propensity to heart disease that is linked with metabolic syndrome.

- When you have the urge to eat, use exercise as one of your enjoyable distractions. Tony, for instance, took a break from the computer, where he was accustomed to eating, to ride an exercise bike at home. Cycling replaced the time when he used to run, without hurting his knees but providing many of the same benefits.
- Strap on a pedometer (you can buy them inexpensively at sporting goods stores or order online from sites such as www.digiwalker .com or www.accusplit.com), and challenge yourself to increase your steps by at least 100 steps each day. Barbara and her husband did, and it worked. They like the competition of seeing which of them has come closest to making their goal of 10,000 steps (five miles) a day. Walking with a pedometer increases motivation because the results are quantifiable; at the same time, it increases your exercise level. Some pedometers even show how many calories you are burning!
- Put on some upbeat music when you take a walk. It will help to keep you going to the beat and provide a distraction so you'll walk for longer.
- Post a weekly activity log on your refrigerator at first to remind you to exercise. Cross it off each day as you do it.
- If you have to miss a day of planned exercise, instead of thinking you have failed, make an appointment with yourself to get exer-

cise the next day. Walking four days a week instead of five is much better than not walking at all.

For many of you, these changes can easily be made on your own. But we know that for some of you these may seem like dramatic or even impossible changes. Because of their importance in changing your gene-based risks, please don't hesitate to seek help from a professional, such as a registered dietitian, licensed mental health professional, physician, or certified personal trainer.

STEP FOUR: FOLLOWING THE PHENOTYPE D DIET

The Phenotype D Diet immediately puts you on the path to losing weight and reducing the many risks of diabetes by turning your food-based weight gain triggers into weight loss triggers with a specific food list, structured meals, and sensible portions. With 45 percent of calories from carbohydrate, 20 percent from protein, and 35 percent from predominantly monounsaturated fat, this diet controls blood glucose and reduces insulin resistance on a cellular level as you lose weight. As a result, you will feel healthier and more energetic and avoid fat as your fate.

Incidentally, one small group of people with type 2 diabetes has a slightly different genetic picture. Weight gain is not a problem for them.

The Phenotype D Diet will change your diet to lose weight and improve your health with the following critical changes:

- Eating a *low-glycemic-index/load* diet
- Including high-fiber carbohydrates daily
- Drinking unsweetened and no-carb beverages
- Including antioxidant foods daily
- Including magnesium foods daily
- And, to reduce heart disease risk:
  - Increasing omega-3 fats relative to omega-6 fats to reduce LDL levels and inflammation
  - Eating more nuts for their role in satiety and lipid profile improvement
  - Eating seafood meals at least two times per week
  - Substituting nonhydrogenated unsaturated fats for saturated fats and trans (partially hydrogenated) fats

However, Phenotype D Focus Foods can limit their cellular damage and improve their condition by enriching their nutrition with vitamin E, vitamin C, selenium, copper, manganese, and magnesium.

Focus Foods

Phenotype D Focus Foods help prevent or treat diabetes and the metabolic syndrome associated with diabetes and related health problems while you're losing weight. All work well with glucose-lowering medications.

High-fiber carbohydrates: High-fiber carbohydrates help normalize blood glucose and insulin levels and lower blood cholesterol. Having a lower *glycemic load,* they provide an advantage over the processed carbohydrates and refined sugars that are such a problem for diabetics. High-fiber carbohydrates also delay stomach emptying, providing you with a feeling of fullness known as *satiety.* Typically, high-fiber foods are also lower in calories from fat and sugar but naturally high in vitamins, minerals, antioxidants, and phytochemicals that boost the nutritional quality of the diet.

The United States is often referred to as the most constipated society. This has nothing to do with attitude but everything to do with the fact that we consume only 14–15 grams of fiber from our food every day versus the needed 20–35+ grams. Fiber sources such as apples, beans and legumes, oatmeal, and other fruits and vegetables are good sources of dietary fiber. For a list of high-fiber foods, see Appendix F.

Two scientific quantifiers of carbohydrates—the *glycemic index* and the *glycemic load*—may be of interest to Phenotype Ds, though you need *not* learn the glycemic values of foods to follow the Phenotype D Diet.

The Glycemic Index and the Glycemic Load

The *glycemic index* is a measure of the body's blood glucose increase, represented by precise scores for carbohydrate foods when they are eaten alone in a portion that provides 50 grams of carbohydrate. Fifty grams can be an enormous quantity, depending on the food item. Fiber content, cooking time, and time of digestion also can affect glycemic index.

The *glycemic load,* on the other hand, is a more comprehensive score. Specifically, the glycemic load reflects two measurements—how much carbohydrate is eaten in an actual serving and how long it takes for that to be digested and released into the bloodstream, which determines the rise in blood glucose. Obviously, in Phenotype Ds, the risk of type 2 diabetes is increased when the glycemic load of the diet is high.

Many weight loss diets base their lists of food to eat or not to eat only on the glycemic index instead of on the glycemic load. This is a skewed process, because the index does not quantify the amount of carbohydrate in a real serving size. For instance, these diets might advise people to limit their intake of carrots due to their relatively high glycemic index score. However, you would have to eat ¾ pound of carrots to reach the 50 grams indicated by the glycemic index. If you look at the glycemic load, carrots receive a much lower score than they do on the glycemic index and are not a problem. In the examples below, looking just at glycemic index, popcorn and carrots have the highest glycemic index. However, when you look at the glycemic load of these examples, only the apple juice is high.

Neither glycemic index nor glycemic load scores exist for meat, poultry, fish, avocados, salad greens, cheese, or eggs, because these foods contain little or no carbohydrate. Nevertheless, good nutrition requires more than protein and fat. Carbohydrates provide fuel for the body and brain, as well

RECOMMENDED GLYCEMIC INDEX VALUES

Low glycemic index foods	Glycemic index of 55 or less
Intermediate glycemic index foods	Glycemic index of 56–69
High glycemic index foods	Glycemic index of 70 or greater

RECOMMENDED GLYCEMIC LOAD VALUES

Low glycemic load foods	Glycemic load of 10 or less
Intermediate glycemic load foods	Glycemic load of 11–19
High glycemic load foods	Glycemic load of 20 or more

GLYCEMIC INDEX VERSUS GLYCEMIC LOAD

Food	Glycemic Index	Glycemic Load
Carrots, ½ cup	110	10
Popcorn, 3 cups	72	8
Apple juice, 1 cup	58	17
Apple, 1 raw	52	8
Kidney beans, 1 cup	42	7

as important nutrients such as fiber, B vitamins, vitamins A, C, and D, and needed minerals such as calcium and iron.

In the Phenotype D Diet, we have already adjusted your food list to provide optimal glycemic index foods. We have also adjusted the carbohydrate level to 45 percent *and* switched from low-fiber to high-fiber carbs to provide an optimal glycemic load. When you follow the number of carbohydrates allowed on the diet and the choices given, using your palm, fist, or thumb to control the amounts, the right glycemic index and load will be maintained and you will lose weight.

Unsweetened beverages: Added sugars, found in beverages such as soft drinks, sports drinks, and fruit drinks significantly increase the amount of processed carbohydrates and excess calories consumed. These drinks may contain as much as 9 to 12 teaspoons of sugar in 12 ounces, and they are liquid calories that don't contribute nutrition or enhance satiety. Instead choose unsweetened and no-carb beverages such as bottled water, diet sodas, and unsweetened tea or coffee, and save your carbs for real food.

Antioxidant foods: A diet containing ample quantities of antioxidants offsets cellular damage. It may even prevent the expression of the genes for diabetes when combined with other Focus Foods. Antioxidants are natural chemicals found in foods that protect the cells from oxidative damage and protect their ability to function normally. The antioxidants vitamin E, vitamin C, selenium, copper, manganese, and magnesium in the diet are beneficial to all diabetics and significantly improve the genetic mitochondrial damage category of diabetes that affects a small percentage of diabetics. Colorful fruits and vegetables are the best sources of antioxidants. The

TOP TWENTY ANTIOXIDANT FOODS

Asparagus	Citrus
Blueberries	Winter squash
Broccoli	Green, red, and orange peppers
Cantaloupe	Strawberries
Carrots	Leafy greens
Nectarines	Watermelon
Papaya	Beets
Peaches	Mangoes
Spinach	Pumpkin
Tomatoes	Cabbage

WAYS TO ADD ANTIOXIDANTS

INSTEAD OF:	USE:
Iceberg lettuce	Romaine, spinach, red leaf, or spring salad mix
Tomato sauce	Vegetable sauce (add shredded carrots or zucchini; see recipe for Vegetable Spaghetti Sauce in Appendix C)
Cole slaw	Cabbage and broccoslaw (bagged in the produce section)
White potatoes	Sweet potatoes

brighter and more intense the produce's color, the more loaded it is with naturally occurring antioxidants.

Magnesium-rich foods: One in three people with diabetes has low magnesium levels, which in turn aggravates carbohydrate intolerance. Adequate magnesium in the diet can improve the delicate balancing act among glucose, insulin, and other hormones.

Coffee: For Phenotype Ds, coffee may be beneficial because there is some indication that it may reduce insulin resistance. Harvard researchers found

MAGNESIUM-RICH FOODS

Trail mix with whole grains such as oatmeal, nuts, and seeds
Oat bran
Chocolate
Halibut
Spinach
Pumpkin seeds
Beans
Nuts
Couscous
Oranges
Grapefruit

that drinking four or more cups of coffee a day is associated with a lower risk of developing type 2 diabetes. Does this mean that if you don't drink coffee, you should start? No. But if you do drink coffee, there's no reason to change your morning coffee ritual or that daily trip to the coffee shop.

Diabetes and metabolic syndrome greatly increase your risk for heart disease. The rest of the Focus Foods are recommended in both the Phenotype C and Phenotype D Diets.

Plant stanol/sterol products such as Take Control Light and Benecol Light spreads or Minute Maid Heart Wise juice: Plant stanols and sterols are found naturally in corn, rice, soybeans, squash, other plants, and vegetable oils. They are chemically related to cholesterol yet very different in that humans absorb them poorly. Consuming products made with sterols or stanols blocks the absorption of both dietary and body-manufactured cholesterol from the intestine into the bloodstream, resulting in a reduction of your total and LDL blood cholesterol. Use these stanols/sterols spreads just like regular butter or margarine, on everything from toast, bagels, and oatmeal to corn on the cob, baked sweet potatoes, and steamed veggies. We recommend the light version of these spreads for their lower calories. There are no reported side effects, and studies have shown that a continuous intake of one to two servings per day can lower total cholesterol by about 10 percent (decreasing without negatively affecting HDL). If you discontinue these products, your total and LDL cholesterol may return to their previous levels. Both products can be used with statin medications or glucose-lowering medications.

Look for Take Control Light and Benecol Light spreads in your grocery with margarines.

Nuts and seeds: Nuts and seeds have a low glycemic load, and portions of 1 to 2 ounces per day have been shown to lower cholesterol by 5 to 15 percent. The improvement in cholesterol results from a synergistic effect among the various powerful ingredients, including fiber, magnesium, folate, protein, monounsaturated fat, and vitamin E. The latest studies credit the "gamma" form of vitamin E in nuts, seeds, and oils, not the "alpha" form found in most vitamin E supplements, for working with other nutrients to lower cholesterol.

We're talking not just peanuts but almonds, walnuts, macadamias, and soy nuts as well. However, this is one item that demands close attention when it comes to portion size. Sesame seeds and pumpkin seeds are also great in the portions recommended in the Food List later in this chapter (see page 161). Nuts and nut butters such as peanut and cashew butter are very healthy, but to include them regularly, something else has to go, because an ounce of nuts is 160 to 180 calories. You'll notice that your NO-TIME and MORE-TIME Menus use them frequently but somewhat sparingly, such as tossed in a salad, mixed with yogurt, or on top of hot cereal.

Seafood: The omega-3 fatty acids eicosapentaenoic acid (EPA) and docosahexaenoic acid (DHA) found in fish help protect the heart in several ways. By decreasing inflammation levels in the arteries, as evidenced in a lower C-reactive protein (CRP) index, they diminish the buildup of arterial plaque, which can break off and result in a heart attack. Omega-3 fatty acids also promote blood vessel elasticity, reduce the formation of blood clots, keep heart rhythms stable, and lower blood triglyceride levels.

People should not overlook the importance of keeping the ratio of omega-6s to omega-3s within a healthy range. When omega-6s overshadow the omega-3s, COX-2 levels go up and inflammation increases. In the United States, unfortunately, the omega-6 intake is estimated to be fifteen to twenty times higher than the omega-3 intake because the typical American diet is full of processed foods. Processed food often contains corn, sunflower, and safflower oils, all thought to be "heart healthy" since they don't increase blood cholesterol, but they are high in omega-6 polyunsaturated fat. You can achieve a better balance and less inflammation by adding more fish and other omega-3 containing foods (such as canola oil, soybeans, walnuts, soybean oil, and flax) to your diet while cutting back some on products with the omega-6 oils.

> C-reactive protein (CRP) is an index of inflammation levels in the arteries. It can be measured by a blood test called a high-sensitivity CRP test (hs-CRP) and is recommended for Phenotype Ds and those with a family history of heart disease, even when their blood cholesterol level is normal.

Olive oil, olives, canola oil: These are great sources of monounsaturated fat and are rich in oleic acid, which has anti-inflammatory actions similar to those of omega-3 oils in fish. When substituted for saturated fat or polyunsaturated fat, monounsaturated fat from olives, olive oil, or canola oil has been shown to lower total cholesterol and lower LDL cholesterol without negatively affecting HDL cholesterol.

What's the big deal about substituting monounsaturated fats for saturated fats and trans fats? See Appendix E.

FOCUS FOOD FREQUENCY

FOOD ITEM	FREQUENCY
High-fiber carbohydrates	At each meal or snack
Unsweetened beverages	Daily
Antioxidant foods	Daily
Magnesium foods	Daily
Coffee	Daily
Benecol Light or Take Control Light or Minute Maid Heart Wise juice	1 tablespoon 1–2 times per day 8 ounces per day
Nuts and seeds	3–4 times per week
Soybean oil, olives, canola oil	Daily as an oil source in salad dressings or in cooking
Seafood	2–3 times per week

Begin with the Phenotype D *FAST TRACK* Two Weeks

With its quick results, the *FAST TRACK* Two Weeks gets you motivated to keep going. The *FAST TRACK* is too severe for achieving long-term changes to your phenotype, but it will jump-start your weight loss. You'll begin to feel leaner, healthier, and sexier within days. It uses the same format as the Phenotype D Diets for men and women below, with the following exceptions:

1. Omit the number of proteins, carbohydrates and fats from the Phenotype D Diet, as **boldfaced** in parentheses in the Meals and Snacks below.
2. Omit the two fist-size 🖐 🖐 portions of "Sweets, Treats, and Alcohol" (see page 163) allowed each week.
3. Take a multivitamin/mineral supplement as well as the recommended additional vitamin C and vitamin E daily (see "Supplements" on page 168).
4. Start Week 3 with the full Phenotype D Diet.

THE PHENOTYPE D DIET FOR WOMEN

Select your foods for each meal and snack from the Food List on page 161. Sample Menus using foods that fit the diet are on page 164.

Meal 1
1 Protein (any fist, ½ fist, or thumb[s] selection)
2 Carbohydrates
1 Fat
Freebie beverages

Meal 2
2 Proteins (1 palm **or** any 2: fist, ½ fist, or thumb[s] selections)
  (omit 1 protein for *FAST TRACK* Two Weeks)
2 Carbohydrates
Freebie vegetables
2 Fats
Freebie beverages

Meal 3
2 Proteins (any 2: fist, ½ fist, or thumb[s] selections)
3 Carbohydrates **(omit 1 carbohydrate for *FAST TRACK* Two Weeks)**
Freebie vegetables
3 Fats **(omit 1 fat for *FAST TRACK* Two Weeks)**
Freebie beverages

Snack
1 Protein (any fist, ½ fist, or thumb[s] selection)
Freebie beverages

THE PHENOTYPE D DIET FOR MEN

Select your foods for each meal and snack from the Food List on page 161. Sample menus using foods that fit the diet are on page 166.

Meal 1
1 Protein (any fist, ½ fist, or thumb[s] selection)
2 Carbohydrates
2 Fats **(omit 1 fat for *FAST TRACK* Two Weeks)**
Freebie beverages

Meal 2
2 Proteins (1 palm **or** any 2: fist, ½ fist, or thumb[s] selections)
  (omit 1 protein for *FAST TRACK* Two Weeks)
3 Carbohydrates **(omit 1 carbohydrate for *FAST TRACK* Two Weeks)**
Freebie vegetables
3 Fats
Freebie beverages

Meal 3
2 Proteins (any 2: fist, ½ fist, or thumb[s] selections)
4 Carbohydrates **(omit 1 carbohydrate for *FAST TRACK* Two Weeks)**
Freebie vegetables
3 Fats
Freebie beverages

Snack
1 Protein (any fist, ½ fist, or thumb[s] selection)
1 Carbohydrate
Freebie beverages

Stopped losing weight? Refer to "How to Deal with Plateaus" on page 28 and reboot your diet with another *FAST TRACK* Two Weeks.

FOOD LIST

Focus Foods are in **bold type.**

How much of each food should you eat? Use your hand as your guide. Eat the amount that you see; that is, the size of your fist, your palm, or your thumb.

  PALM

  FIST

  THUMB

Protein Sources

 Seafood. Poultry without skin, or lean cuts of meat such as loin, round, or cutlets of beef, pork, ham, veal, venison, lamb, etc.; cook by steaming, sautéing, broiling, or grilling. Meat alternative (tofu, tempeh, or other soy product)

 Skim milk, buttermilk, evaporated skim milk, low-fat yogurt, low-fat cottage cheese, calcium fortified soy milk, **eggs such as Eggland's Best Eggs that are rich in omega-3 fatty acids (100 mg per egg),** ricotta cheese (fat free)

½ **Edamame, garbanzo, pinto, kidney, black, lima, or white beans; split, black-eyed, or field peas; lentils**

  Parmigiano-Reggiano, grana padana, string cheese, Neufchâtel (reduced-fat cream cheese), soy cheese, **peanut butter, almond butter or other nut butters, walnuts, almonds, Brazil nuts, cashews, chestnuts, hazelnuts, macadamia nuts, mixed nuts, peanuts, pecans, pine nuts, pistachios, soy nuts, pumpkin seeds, sunflower seeds**

 Swiss, Cheddar, mozzarella, Romano, colby, feta, Gorgonzola, goat, or Monterey Jack cheese

Carbohydrate Sources

Whole grain bread, corn tortilla, whole wheat tortilla, whole grain English muffin or bagel, whole wheat pita or ½ round whole grain lavash, whole grain crackers, polenta, focaccia bread, corn bread, whole grain muffins, whole grain waffles or pancakes

Popped popcorn

High-fiber cereal, muesli

Apple, banana, berries, carambola (star fruit), cherries, citrus, grapes, kiwi fruit, melon, mango, nectarine, peach, pear, pineapple, plum

100% fruit juice, plain, calcium-fortified, or stanol/sterol-fortified (limit to once a day)

½ Grits; oatmeal; Wheatena; couscous, whole wheat pasta, pasta with at least 2 grams of fiber per serving; brown rice or other whole grain; garbanzo, pinto, kidney, black, lima, or white beans; split, black-eyed, or field peas; lentils; edamame; corn; green peas; potatoes with skin; acorn or butternut squash; sweet potatoes or yams; plantain

Dried fruit such as raisins, cherries, blueberries, apricots, plums, figs, etc.

Flaxseed meal, wheat germ

> Check out the *Freebie* list for lots of veggies, including salad greens, tomatoes, carrots, etc., that you don't have to limit.

Fat Sources

MONOUNSATURATED FATS

Avocado, olives, hummus, almonds, Brazil nuts, cashews, chestnuts, hazelnuts, macadamia nuts, mixed nuts, peanuts, pecans, pine nuts, pistachios, soy nuts, walnuts, pumpkin seeds, safflower seeds, sesame seeds, sunflower seeds

Olive oil, canola oil, peanut oil, tahini, low-trans-fat margarines such as Olivio

POLYUNSATURATED FATS

🥄 🥄 **Benecol Light or Take Control Light spread,** salad dressing, light margarine, light mayonnaise, light salad dressing, low-trans-fat margarines such as Smart Balance

🥄 Benecol or Take Control spread, corn oil, safflower oil, soybean oil, sesame oil, sunflower oil, tartar sauce, salad dressing

Freebies

Beverages: Coffee, tea or diet soft drinks, club soda, carbonated or mineral water

Veggies: Artichoke, artichoke hearts, arugula, asparagus, bean sprouts, beets, Bibb lettuce, broccoli, Brussels sprouts, carrots, cauliflower, cabbage, celery, collard greens, cucumber, endive, eggplant, escarole, green beans, green onions or scallions, green, red, or yellow pepper, kale, kohlrabi, leeks, lettuce, mixed greens, mesclun, mushrooms, mustard greens, okra, onions, pea pods, radishes, romaine, spinach, summer squash, tomato, turnips, turnip greens, water chestnuts, zucchini

Miscellaneous: Broth or bouillon, ketchup, horseradish, lemon juice, lime juice, mustard, pickles, soy sauce, taco sauce, salsa, vinegars, garlic, fresh or dried herbs, pimento, spices, red wine used in cooking, Worcestershire sauce, sugar substitutes

Sweets, Treats, and Alcohol

The Phenotype D Diet gives you two fists 👊 👊 of your choice per week to use as you desire. These treats are already calculated into your diet.

Whether it's a new Italian cheese, the neighbor's Super Bowl party, or a tempting new restaurant down the street, the two fist-size portions of treats weekly keep you in the real world of eating and enjoying food. To keep glucose-wreaked havoc to a minimum, we recommend that Phenotype Ds not eat both fists of goodies at once. But you can still indulge your passion for chocolate almond ice cream gradually over the seven days. That's the beauty of it—it's your choice.

> To use the two fists 👊 👊 as treats, you don't have to subtract anything from the Phenotype D Diet.

Don't forget, alcohol can wreak havoc on your blood triglyceride level. So if you tend to have high triglycerides, consider limiting or even omitting alcohol. Alcohol's love-hate relationship with many drugs can also be a big issue. Interactions can vary from inconsequential to devastating, so if you take *any* prescription or over-the-counter (OTC) drugs, be sure to discuss the use of alcohol with your pharmacist and health care provider.

SAMPLE MENUS

On days when you're rushed, use the NO-TIME Menus. MORE-TIME Menus are for days when you can cook leisurely. The menus are also meant to serve as a guide for eating out.

NO-TIME Menu D for Women

MEAL 1

 Hard-cooked egg

 Oatmeal toast with:

  Benecol Light or Take Control Light

 Pink grapefruit half

Coffee or other *Freebie* beverages

> Look for Take Control Light and Benecol Light spreads in your grocery with margarines.

MEAL 2

Roasted Mozzarella-and-Spinach-Topped Portobellos (see NO-TIME Recipes in Appendix C)

Spiced Carrot-Raisin Salad (see NO-TIME Recipes in Appendix C)

Freebie vegetables

Mango tea or other *Freebie* beverages

MEAL 3

🖐 Susan's Superquick Turkey Chili (see NO-TIME Recipes in Appendix C)

🖐 Parmesan-Topped Broccoli (see NO-TIME Recipes in Appendix C)

Freebie vegetables

Diet soda with lemon or other *Freebie* beverages

SNACK

🖐 Key lime pie yogurt or any flavor that is low-fat and low-sugar or sugar free

MORE-TIME Menu D for Women

MEAL 1

Southwest breakfast burrito with:

🥟 Whole wheat tortilla

🖐 Scrambled egg (such as Eggland's Best)

½ 🖐 Refried beans (low-fat or fat free)

Freebie Salsa

Coffee or other *Freebie* beverages

MEAL 2

🖐 Lentil-Vegetable Soup (see MORE-TIME Recipes in Appendix C) with:

👍 👍 Grana padana cheese

Freebie vegetables

Spiced raspberry tea or other *Freebie* beverages

MEAL 3

Easy Onion Chicken (see MORE-TIME Recipes in Appendix C)

Wild rice

Freebie Sautéed baby spinach with garlic and   pine nuts

Golden pineapple

Freebie vegetables

Tea, coffee or other *Freebie* beverages

SNACK

Vanilla soy milk

NO-TIME Menu D for Men

MEAL 1

Hard-cooked egg

Oatmeal toast with:

   Benecol Light or Take Control Light

Pink grapefruit half

Coffee or other *Freebie* beverages

> Look for Take Control Light and Benecol Light spreads in your grocery with margarines.

MEAL 2

Roasted Mozzarella-and-Spinach-Topped Portobellos (see NO-TIME recipes in Appendix C)

Spiced Carrot-Raisin Salad (see NO-TIME Recipes in Appendix C)

Seven-grain roll with   Benecol Light or Take Control Light spread

Freebie vegetables

Mango tea or other *Freebie* beverages

MEAL 3

Susan's Superquick Turkey Chili (see NO-TIME Recipes in Appendix C) with:

Baked tortilla chips

Parmesan-Topped Broccoli (see NO-TIME Recipes in Appendix C)

Freebie vegetables

Diet soda with lemon or other *Freebie* beverages

SNACK

Key lime pie yogurt or any flavor that is low-fat and low-sugar or sugar free

Banana

MORE-TIME Menu D for Men

MEAL 1

Southwest breakfast burrito with:

Whole wheat tortilla

Scrambled egg (such as Eggland's Best)

½ Refried beans (low-fat or fat free)

Freebie Salsa

Coffee or other *Freebie* beverages

MEAL 2

Lentil-Vegetable Soup (see MORE-TIME Recipes in Appendix C) with:

Grana padana cheese

Slice of warm pumpernickel raisin bread with Take Control Light or Benecol Light spread

Freebie vegetables

Spiced raspberry tea or other *Freebie* beverages

MEAL 3

Easy Onion Chicken (see MORE-TIME Recipes in Appendix C)

½ Wild rice

Freebie Sautéed baby spinach with garlic and pine nuts

Golden pineapple

Freebie vegetables

Tea, coffee, or other *Freebie* beverages

SNACK

Banana nut bread with:

Neufchâtel cream cheese (low-fat)

Supplements

Chromium: The mineral chromium, a catalyst of sorts, helps insulin carry glucose from the breakdown of food into the cells for use as energy. Chromium supplements may reduce insulin resistance and improve blood sugar control in people with type 2 diabetes.

Lipoic acid (alpha-lipoic acid, or ALA): Lipoic acid is a vitamin-like substance with antioxidant properties. It is now being explored for other benefits, which include lowering blood sugar levels and reducing oxidative stress and inflammation in people with type 2 diabetes.

Bilberry: Often called the European blueberry, bilberry is very similar to the American blueberry or huckleberry. Bilberry contains phytochemicals called *anthocyanosides*. Bilberry lowers blood sugar levels in people with diabetes who are taking glucose-lowering medications. Its anthocyanosides strengthen the walls of blood vessels and reduce inflammation, particularly in the eyes.

Omega-3 fatty acids: These are fats such as eicosapentaenoic acid (EPA) and docosahexaenoic acid (DHA), which are common in the oils of fish. If you do not eat fish, consider taking a fish oil supplement. Taking supplements containing omega-3 fatty acids, up to 1 gram per day, has been shown to reduce blood triglyceride levels, raise HDL levels, act as blood thinners, reduce homocysteine levels, and have anti-inflammatory effects.

Choose a supplement that, taken three times a day, provides a **total** of approximately 900 mg per day of EPA and DHA. Most 1,000 mg capsules contain 180 mg EPA and 120 mg DHA each. At these recommended doses, side effects such as fishy aftertaste, stomach distress, or a rise in LDL cholesterol are minimal. As doses increase above these recommended levels, the side effects increase. *If you are taking prescription blood thinners such as warfarin (Coumadin) or heparin or are expecting to undergo surgery, ask your physician before taking fish oil supplements.*

Psyllium (such as Metamucil): Psyllium is a high-fiber treatment for constipation. It's sold over the counter as a laxative in pill, powder, and wafer form and as an ingredient in the breakfast cereal Bran Buds. As with any fiber source, whether food or supplement, you must drink more water when taking it and add the fiber to your diet slowly. Ten to 15 grams of psyllium a day reduces glucose load and blood sugar levels by 12 percent.

SUPPLEMENT RECOMMENDATIONS AND DOSES

SUPPLEMENT	DOSE
Multivitamin/mineral	Daily
Vitamin C	250 mg daily

(continued on next page)

SUPPLEMENT	DOSE
Vitamin E	200 IU mixed tocopherols for women daily; 400 IU mixed tocopherols for men daily
Chromium	500–1,000 micrograms (µg) daily; check to see how much is in your daily multivitamin/mineral supplement
Lipoic acid	300 to 600 mg daily in two to three divided doses
Bilberry	120–240 mg twice daily
Omega-3 or fish oil supplements	The latest American Heart Association recommendations are: 2–4 grams of supplemental fish oil daily if you have high blood triglycerides above 200 mg/dl as in metabolic syndrome; to get this amount, take two 1,000 mg fish oil capsule three times per day with meals, since most 1,000 mg capsules contain only 180 mg EPA and 120 mg DHA each
Psyllium	1 round teaspoon (3–4 grams) taken 1–3 times daily; start at the lowest dose and increase your water intake by 8 oz for each teaspoon used; or take 2–4 wafers providing 3 grams each

The Phenotype D Maintenance Diet

Remember when you started on the Phenotype D Diet? In a few days, something inside just seemed to click and you began to lose weight, feel better, and feel healthier. That will not change. When you reach your weight goal, you are ready to move on to the Phenotype D Maintenance Diet. The diet has the same backbone Focus Foods. Still tailored to your genetic blueprint, it will keep you satisfied and your weight constant. Tony, as an example, was able to go out to dinner more frequently, even indulge in an occasional sweet, and still keep his blood glucose under control, as long as he concentrated on the low-glycemic-load foods and high-fiber carbs recommended in the diet. Of course, a high level of physical activity or exercise is the single best predictor of keeping lost weight off. So keep moving!

THE PHENOTYPE D MAINTENANCE DIET FOR WOMEN

Meal 1
1 Protein (any fist, ½ fist, or thumb[s] selection)
2 Carbohydrates
1 Fat
Freebie beverages

Meal 2
2 Proteins (1 palm **or** any 2: fist, ½ fist, or thumb[s] selections)
2 Carbohydrates
Freebie vegetables
3 Fats
Freebie beverages

Meal 3
2 Proteins (any 2: fist, ½ fist, or thumb[s] selections)
3 Carbohydrates
Freebie vegetables
3 Fats
Freebie beverages

Snack
1 Protein (any fist, ½ fist, or thumb[s] selection)
1 Carbohydrate
Freebie beverages

THE PHENOTYPE D
MAINTENANCE DIET FOR MEN

Meal 1
2 Proteins (any fist, ½ fist, or thumb[s] selection)
2 Carbohydrates
2 Fats
Freebie beverages

Meal 2
2 Proteins (1 palm **or** any 2: fist, ½ fist, or thumb[s] selections)
3 Carbohydrates
Freebie vegetables
3 Fats
Freebie beverages

Meal 3
2 Proteins (any 2: fist, ½ fist, or thumb[s] selections)
4 Carbohydrates
Freebie vegetables
4 Fats
Freebie beverages

Snack
2 Proteins (any fist, ½ fist, or thumb[s] selection)
1 Carbohydrate
1 Fat
Freebie beverages

CHAPTER 8

The Phenotype E Diet

OUTSMARTING EMOTIONAL
EATING–LINKED WEIGHT GAIN

Tamara's Story

"I can't wait until he falls asleep in the recliner and starts to snore, because I know he's not watching and I can eat anything I want."

Throughout most of Tamara's thirty-year marriage, her husband has made hurtful comments about her weight. Tamara felt that he constantly watched what she ate, and it made her feel deprived. She told us that he regularly accused her of "cheating" on her diet and didn't understand why she couldn't just "stick to it" to lose the pounds. Tamara believed that his negative taunting increased her emotional eating and sabotaged her weight loss. As she put it, "It's one thing to have your girlfriends talk about how you look, but when the person you love makes degrading comments, it hurts—and it hurts a lot. It has affected my self-esteem and self-confidence."

His constant teasing and bullying drove Tamara into a desperate cycle of eating deprivation followed by indulgence. Her typical day began with coffee in the car, then gave way to leftover pizza at lunch and a big meal in the evening, followed by the "I'll show you" eating late at night. Tamara said, "I usually grab a bag of potato chips or some other salty carb whenever I'm depressed, and then I'm depressed because I'm eating. I feel fat and frustrated." She was tired and had little energy left for her three children and an active schedule that included working part time, pursuing her master's degree, and volunteering at church. Tamara felt her life and health were in a downward spiral fueled by guilt.

When 5'4" Tamara tipped the scales at 190 pounds, she decided the emotional eating had to stop. To regain control over her intake as well as put a stop to the onslaught of upsetting comments, she began the Phenotype E Diet. Tamara has kept a private journal since she was a child to reflect, often to vent or clarify her innermost thoughts and feelings. Continuing it as part of the Phenotype E Food Record process, she had no problem recognizing her pattern of revenge eating.

After five weeks of following the diet, Tamara had lost 12 pounds and gained more energy. An avid tennis player, she started noticing a difference in her stamina during matches. "I like the feeling of control over what I'm doing," she wrote.

If you are overweight and a Phenotype E, you answered "yes" to some of these statements in the Phenotype Assessment:

- I eat more when I'm sad, happy, lonely, upset, bored, or stressed.
- I tend to overeat more when I'm alone or in big groups, such as at parties.
- There are times when I feel my eating is hard to control.
- I eat to calm my feelings.
- I sometimes feel ashamed of my eating.

STEP ONE: UNDERSTANDING YOUR PHENOTYPE

Phenotype Es gain weight as a result of emotional eating. If you and/or family members treat hassles and hurt with quantities of food or are prone to depression, you are a Phenotype E. Emotional eaters eat when they are sad, hurt, lonely, bored, stressed, tired, or dreading a difficult task. It is very common. Even Sarah Ferguson, the Duchess of York, has discussed her emotional eating on national television.

Your Desire for Food Is Emotionally Driven, Not Hunger Driven

For Phenotype Es, *eating is more about emotions and less about food.* Emotional eating leads to weight gain because eating doesn't result from hunger signals but erupts in response to difficult feelings and stressful situations. Study after study correlates stress and depression with unwanted weight. *Preventive Medicine* reported a higher body mass index (BMI) (a measure of body fatness based on height and weight) among stress eaters, particularly women. The stress eaters tended to eat sausages, hamburgers, pizza, and chocolate more frequently than non–stress eaters. The best predictors of stress eating among men were being single or divorced, a long history of unemployment, and a low level of education. Among women, the best predictor of stress eating was a lack of emotional support. *Obesity Research* found stress and depression to be the major predictors of emotional eating in overweight women.

There is a scientific reason why you use food to cope with life's events, to mask difficult feelings, or to bridge stressful situations. Yes, this classic Phenotype E response has a physiological basis. You are attempting to bring your complicated body chemistry under control. Mood changes can reflect fluctuating blood glucose levels, uneven supplies of body fuel that result from skipping meals or having the wrong mix of protein, carbohydrate, and fat. In addition, mental well-being requires adequate quantities of *neurotransmitters*, chemicals that transmit messages between nerves in the brain. It also requires the cell-surface receptors to transmit them. So inadequate quantities of neurotransmitters or receptors for neurotransmitters, including serotonin, are involved in mood instability. Thus, the emotional eating response has a genetic basis. It is also partly learned. When you add stressful situations to the mix, stress creates a surge of cortisol, a steroid hormone. Together, decreased serotonin and increased cortisol send an "eat carbohydrate" message to the brain. For Phenotype Es, the message can be an invitation to overeat.

Food Affects Your Brain Chemicals

When you eat carbohydrate, your blood glucose levels rise and trigger the release of insulin. Insulin causes the large neutral amino acids (LNAAs)—tyrosine, phenylalanine, leucine, and isoleucine—to be taken up into muscle. At the same time, another LNAA, tryptophan, competes with these other LNAAs for the same transport molecule to get into the brain. Consuming a meal of pure carbohydrate increases the ratio of tryptophan to these other LNAAs in the blood. Hence, more tryptophan makes its way to the brain, where it converts to serotonin.

That's why Phenotype Es reach for refined sugars and carbohydrates, because the serotonin it produces contributes to making them feel better. The problem is that the "high" is brief. Their blood sugar level soon plummets, and so does their energy level. For emotional eaters, this cycle re-creates the need to eat, for both physiological and emotional reasons. The physiological need is triggered by the fall in blood sugar, and the emotional need is triggered by the stress or the emotional reaction to the stress. These blood sugar fluctuations acutally increase the stress level that triggered the eating to start with. Emotional eaters overeat for comfort, not hunger.

Protein in food affects the conversion of tryptophan to serotonin, since protein provides the competing LNAA to prevent tryptophan from crossing into the brain. Nevertheless, research indicates that a diet that overall is high in carbohydrate helps to improve moods.

High-fat foods deliver their own "feel-good" response by releasing endorphins, the same mood-enhancing neurochemicals released during exercise, and satisfying emotional cravings. Endorphins are morphinelike chemicals that exert analgesic effects by binding to opiate receptors on brain cells and increasing the pain threshold. They produce a powerful pleasure sensation. Cravings for high-fat foods correspond to the shift in hormones around puberty. Before puberty, children crave mostly sugar as a preferred food taste. Around puberty, young men begin to prefer the combination of protein and fat, spurred by their need to build muscle. Young women seek out sugar-fat combos, driven by estrogen to store fat and prepare for possible pregnancy. These preferences persist into adulthood. Phenotype E men favor burgers or pizza, while phenotype E women desire sugar-fat combinations. That's why chocolate is their number one food craving. Because of its sugar content, chocolate can increase brain serotonin levels and, due to its fat content, increase endorphins at the same time. This combination of brain chemicals is often described as "optimal brain happiness." For both genders, these food combos can temporarily improve mood, but in excess amounts they layer on the weight.

Better Food Choices Sustain Better Emotions

The trick for Phenotype Es is not just to elevate serotonin but also to create a steady glucose level. We recommend a combination of high-fiber carbohydrates and protein, combined with antioxidant-rich produce. These foods take longer to digest than simple sugars and produce a more steady-state blood glucose level, reducing the highs and lows caused by refined carbs alone. This sustains the feeling of energy emotional eaters desire.

As a Phenotype E, you must first recognize the connection between emotion and food, then work vigilantly to deliver more even and consis-

---

Some emotional eaters are actually depressed and may not know it. The latest estimate is that more than 20 million Americans are depressed and half are undiagnosed. The current thinking is that 50 percent of depression is brought on by negative life events and 50 percent is based on your genetics. If you know you have a family history of mood disorders such as depression, or if you eat your way through difficult situations, you should take the following Depression Quiz.

HOW HIGH IS YOUR DEPRESSION RISK?
PLEASE ANSWER THE FOLLOWING QUESTIONS.

1. Are activities that you have always found pleasurable no longer enjoyable?
2. Do you feel tired all the time without any apparent reason?
3. Do you sleep more than usual or have insomnia?
4. Do you feel like eating all the time, especially sweets, or has your appetite decreased significantly?
5. Do tasks that used to seem simple now seem very difficult?
6. Are you avoiding friends and crowds?
7. Are you having a very hard time getting over a loss or trauma in your life?
8. Are you feeling hopeless and worthless, as though life is not worth living?
9. Are you unable to go to work or keep up with responsibilities that are part of your daily life because you feel bad and don't know why?

If you answered yes to four or more of these questions, and especially if you answered yes to Question 8, it's time to see your physician or a mental health professional. Depression is not a character flaw; it's a very treatable medical condition. Research has shown that talk therapy and medication work together to correct the neurotransmitter changes associated with depression, improve your mood, and help you deal with stressful life events. A therapist or counselor, psychologist, or psychiatrist can provide the right combination of talk therapy and medication that is most effective in dealing with depression or other mood disorders.

Depression is seen more in women than in men and tends to recur periodically. Stressful events can precipitate or aggravate an episode in someone who has a family history of depression. Because the Phenotype E Diet is designed to maximize foods' effect on your mood, you can boost the effectiveness of any treatment you receive for depression by following the Phenotype E guidelines in this chapter.

tent supplies of nutrients to your system, to support your emotional well-being. It is time to redirect your emotions with positive food choices and positive behaviors. By following the Phenotype E Diet and changing your triggers, you can actually minimize the chemicals that exacerbate emotional upheaval. It follows that with less emotional upheaval, you'll be less apt to overeat.

STEP TWO: KEEPING A FOOD RECORD

Keeping a Food Record is a helpful technique for all phenotypes, but it is *critical* for Phenotype Es because food isn't your problem; emotions are. Writing will expose that as an emotional eater you eat for reasons other than hunger. Don't think you can skip this step!

A Food Record will help you identify the fascinating and often painful connection between eating and mood. For instance, stress is often behind Phenotype E eating habits. You may have noticed this when you took the Weight Trigger Quiz. Stress is the number one trigger for many Phenotype Es. Not only will an eating log help you lose weight more steadily and keep it off, writing will help vent complex emotions and determine where you need to make changes elsewhere in your life.

If you have to write down what and when you eat, then see it in print, it's easier to understand what made you feel like eating, be it stress, emotions, or both. And, it will make you more accountable for your actions. Our clients find they begin to think twice before downing that pint of Ben & Jerry's or nose-diving into a big bag of M&Ms. Until you see your actions in black and white, it's very difficult, if not impossible, to change triggers. To get you started, on the next page is an example of a Food Record to copy or create in a journal you purchase.

This isn't a time to delude yourself. Inventory everything you swallow, meal after meal, day after day. Your Food Record should include when you eat, what you eat, how much you eat, and how you're feeling at the time. Describe what is going on deep inside *you*—not your spouse, not your boss, not your coworkers, and not your kids. If you aren't truthful with yourself, you won't see the pattern between the mood you're in and the food you eat, so keep your Food Record in a safe, private place and be brutally honest with yourself. This is not only eye-opening, it's life-changing work you're doing.

After you have kept your Food Record for about a week, take some time and study what you have written. Do you see a pattern? What causes your emotions? What foods go along with them? The answers may be shocking or embarrassing at first. Please stick with the Food Record. The payoff will be a healthier, happier, and more empowered you.

EMOTIONAL EATING FOOD RECORD

Date/Time	Location	Food/Beverages Consumed	Amount	Feelings	Degree of Hunger

Use the following scale for degree of hunger: 0 = famished, 5–6 = satisfied, 10 = stuffed

Nick's Story

"Food is love, baby, and I'm Italian."

"I am my biggest problem," admitted Nick, a 57-year-old, 5'7", 303-pound Italian, who had tried them all—diets, that is. He loves to eat, and he loves to cook for his family and friends, demonstrating his affection with fabulous cuisine. He is also very busy. "I have too much to do to record what I eat!" he announced when he began the Phenotype E Diet.

As the owner of three hair salons, Nick said he was constantly on the move—working with stylists, managing vendors, and running day-to-day operations. His downtime was almost nonexistent. "When I get home at the end of the day, I feel like I deserve a reward, so I have a nice dinner and several glasses of fine wine. It helps me relax and deal with the stress."

However, emotional eating associated with stress was significantly jeopardizing his health. Overeating, over time, led Nick to gain a tremendous amount of weight and required him to take several daily drugs, including Lipitor for his cholesterol level.

Yet for the first several weeks of attempting the Phenotype E Diet, Nick didn't follow the concept of eating every two to three hours, nor did he record what he ate. Nick even asked his wife to do his "homework" and tell him how to correct his eating habits. He probably asked her to keep a journal, too! Luckily, she refused.

Finally, Nick began keeping the Food Record. Whenever he had food cravings, he'd ask himself, "Is my desire hunger or habit?" At this point, Nick was facing the emotional issues entangled with his eating and giving himself permission to explore his habits and thoughts.

A month into the program, Nick shared from his Food Record. "I spent a lot of time thinking about what you said. Men have a fear of losing weight. We are creatures of habit and fear that we'll have to change. I realized that I needed to take control of something that has had control of me for years and years. It's been hard for me to feel good about myself when I know I could do better. Inside, men know their successes and failures—things they don't tell anyone else.

"I have to look at dieting the way I look at my businesses; that is, by setting a goal and working towards it. I used to think I knew it all, and when people would say to me, 'I'll pray for you,' I would say, 'Don't pray for me, pray for yourself.' I was an arrogant know-it-all. Over the years, that attitude has definitely changed. But I still face the issues with food, particularly when I'm stressed, which is most of the time."

Thinking of his weight as a business gave Nick another helpful idea for *dealing with stress. He decided to set aside a "worry time" in the evening to think about the issues on his mind for a set interval of time and then let them go.*

Nick soon discovered he felt more energized when he ate every three hours, although planning and timing meals was a struggle at first. When food is around, he still has the urge to eat it. "The other night my wife made meatballs, and two of them jumped right out of the bowl into my mouth," he wrote. Nick continues to struggle with his emotions, but that's okay. He's a Phenotype E, and it's expected. On the other hand, he is making progress and has already lost 17 pounds. He wants to lose 50 by next summer for his overseas trip.

Mimi's Story

"I'm not hungry, just bored."

"I sit at the computer in my home office ten hours a day doing the books for our businesses, and I eat from boredom. Most of the time I don't even realize that I'm doing it. I'm not hungry—it's just habit," Mimi wrote. This habit fed the 5'7" redhead up to 253 pounds.

Keeping a Food Record each time she ate, Mimi rated her hunger levels from 0 to 10, with 0 being famished and 10 as though she had just eaten Thanksgiving dinner. As she looked over what she had written, Mimi noticed that most of her hunger ratings were only 5 or 6. This gave Mimi her "Ah-ha!" moment. She recognized that her eating must be emotionally based.

To replace her eating response, we asked Mimi to set the timer on her computer to alert her to take a stretch break every hour or two—not to eat but to get up, clear her head, drink a glass of water, and walk outside for a few minutes. She found this really helped break her habit of eating to alleviate the monotony.

PREEMPT YOUR EATING RESPONSE WITH THE FOUR Ds

Once you recognize the emotions that are leading you to eat, as Tamara, Nick, and Mimi did, you can change your reaction. To preempt the immediate eating that is literally a "gut reaction" to emotion, our clients and patients have found the **Four Ds** helpful.

- **Deep breathing:** Take ten slow, deep breaths in succession: breathe in to a count of ten, hold for a count of ten, and breathe out slowly to a count of ten.
- **Delay:** Wait at least ten minutes before eating; then see if you still feel like eating.
- **Drink water, coffee, or tea:** Have a glass of water or drink something hot, such as tea or coffee. Drinking helps satisfy the desire to eat.
- **Distraction:** Tailor your distractions to the source of the emotion. If it's stress that habitually makes you eat, schedule a "worry time" as Nick did, or do a mechanical task such as pulling weeds or trimming shrubs to help clear your mind. If it's boredom, commit to a new and stimulating objective. If it's loneliness, call a friend or volunteer at a shelter or library. If you're angry, get physical and go for a brisk walk or clean a closet. Make a list of enjoyable or mechanical distractions you can do instead of eating, such as listening to music, gardening, doing laundry, playing your guitar or piano, cooking a meal for a sick friend, playing with a pet, or sending or answering e-mail.

Rachel's Story

"I have a burning obsession for chocolate."

Are you a card-carrying member of the 24/7 we-never-stop society? Then you'll relate to Rachel, a legal nurse consultant who juggles long hours of research with one hand and quality time with her family with the other. Everyday around 3 to 4 P.M., Rachel used to reach for some type of chocolate, typically peanut M&Ms. Rachel admitted that there were many days when she had a "burning obsession for chocolate."

Sound familiar? This is a typical Phenotype E trend. Rachel's chocolate routine was her way of maintaining a hectic pace and coping with the work-related frustration that went with it.

When Rachel closely analyzed the Food Record she began when she undertook the Phenotype E Diet, she noticed she really wasn't eating much all day—just coffee and maybe a piece of toast for breakfast and generally no lunch unless she met a client. No wonder she was tired. One can't live on MEMs alone.

Rachel recognized that she needed a way to forestall the stress eating, which was most likely to happen in midafternoon or evening, as it does for most emotional eaters. To spread out the calorie intake, she began fueling her body earlier, more often, and more healthfully during the day. She used the Four Ds to deal with her afternoon surge of emotions.

STEP THREE: DEVELOPING POSITIVE NONFOOD WEIGHT LOSS TRIGGERS

Remember that when it comes to weight, your genetics and family history load the gun but ultimately your routines pull the trigger—negatively, toward weight gain, or positively, toward weight loss. The Phenotype E Diet detailed later in this chapter changes the three food-related negative triggers from the Weight Trigger Quiz into positive triggers: best food choices, structured meals, and sensible portions.

How did you score on the Weight Trigger Quiz's nonfood categories: "Stress," "No Regular Exercise," and "Increasingly Sedentary Lifestyle"? Nick answered "true" to eight out of ten questions in the "Stress" category. Too much screen time made Mimi's sedentary lifestyle her main trigger. Neither they nor Rachel got regular exercise.

When moving from negative to positive triggers in these categories, make "deliberate changes," not perfection, your goal. As an example, one of Nick's deliberate changes was beginning to swim. A positive trigger, exercise empowered his phenotype, reinforcing his new eating habits with more efficient metabolism and improved mood. When new triggers kick in, eating patterns change and weight loss happens easily. "This diet is so powerful. I had no idea," Nick wrote. "It's more than weight loss—a lot more. Yesterday I was standing on tile for twelve hours and my legs didn't ache. Then I slept four hours, woke up for a few minutes, and slept three hours more. For someone who has only been sleeping maybe a total of four hours for years, this is big."

We recommend making one change at a time and letting it become a habit before you start the next change. It typically takes three to four weeks for a change to become part of your life. Set nonfood incentives, and reward yourself as you progress. Have a look at the following strategies for turning off your greatest weight gain triggers.

Reduce Your Stress

When examining your key tendencies of emotional eating in your Phenotype E Food Record, you will notice that nervous tension usually makes you reach for food—and lots of it. For example, Nick ate ice cream after every sales meeting to help him relax. Impulses such as these are driven by cortisol, the stress hormone. On the Phenotype E Diet you won't need to stress eat to feel better, because the diet will do the job of keeping you satisfied—without adding weight. Even though the diet changes your eating behaviors by taking charge of when and what you eat, you must still deal with the emotional and stressful issues that have been part of your eating ritual and history for a long time. By dealing with both, you are less likely to let emotional upsets cause a lapse in your diet. But you do need some positive strategies to help you deal with stress, which is the number one cause of diet relapses.

- Every time you feel your emotions getting the better of you, implement the Four Ds that Rachel and Tamara used (See page 182). Create a list of enjoyable distractions, other than food, and use them.
- Set aside a regular worry time. When stress tempts you to overeat or keeps you awake, put the thoughts aside until your scheduled worry time.
- If you are overcommitted, decrease the number of your obligations so you can make more time for yourself.
- If you do lapse, please don't throw in the towel. Adjust your attitude from "I blew the diet" to "One mistake is not a big problem—I am committed to this diet and losing weight with this diet."
- Supersized portions are one of the greatest recent changes contributing to weight gain in the United States, and Phenotype Es are particularly vulnerable because they are easily stressed. When you're stressed, having large portions of food available makes it more likely that you will overeat. As explained in "Understanding Your Phenotype" (page 174), consuming bigger portions makes it feel as if you are treating your emotions, but it actually only increases your stress level and perpetuates your emotional eating pattern. Even though it may cost slightly more, buy foods packaged in single portions to reduce the chances of overeating.

- Make eating a conscious and deliberate event, not something you do when you're stressed. If you eat while driving, watching TV, working at the computer, or doing other activities, you're less likely to feel satisfied and more likely to overindulge. You may not even be aware of what or how much you're eating. Your Food Record can help you here, too. It's hard to eat, write, and drive at the same time!

Develop an Active Lifestyle

Every time Charles, a Phenotype E client, watched TV, he wanted a snack, too, so off to the kitchen he went, hungry or not. It wasn't the food that drew him but the stress-releasing comfort of the ritual. Charles needed strategies to prevent what had become a hand-to-mouth habit to accompany sitting still, just as you may. You have to interrupt the habit with some other motion, such as squeezing a rubber stress ball, drinking a noncalorie drink, or chewing sugarless gum. In addition, a deliberate change toward more activity is needed.

- Turn off the television or computer at least three nights a week and plan other activities.
- Take regular breaks, as Mimi does, to stretch and drink water.
- Walk everywhere you can, even if it's upstairs to eat lunch or down the hall to the water cooler. Get up and move.
- Schedule mini-outings into your day. Mimi made a deliberate change in her workday, walking to the coffee shop and getting a skinny latte every workday around 3 or 3:30 P.M. to avoid the afternoon slump she typically faced at her desk. She got in some walking and a Focus Food serving of skim milk too.

Exercise Regularly

Exercise deflates stress, prevents boredom, and revs up metabolism for hours after the activity. It also produces endorphins, brain chemicals that help to improve mood. For emotional eaters, a daily workout will put emotions on a more even keel. Nick, our star example, was not comfortable going to a gym at 300-plus pounds, but since he had a pool, he hired a trainer to design a water workout ten minutes a day, three to four times a week. He also began swimming at night to relax. He now swims for 30 minutes every morning.

- When you have the urge to eat, use exercise as one of your enjoyable distractions. In other words, keep trying activities until you find an exercise you enjoy or will do routinely.

- Add frequent short bouts of exercise, such as 10 minutes at a time. Ten minutes several times a day add up and break the routine of reaching for food. Most people can walk away from their desk and go somewhere—anywhere—to add activity during a long work-day. Put on your pedometer (see below) and walk around your building or block and watch the steps add up.
- Buy a pedometer (good sources are www.accusplit.com, Target stores, and www.digiwalker.com) and wear it daily so you can see how far you currently walk. Set a goal to increase your distance by at least 100 steps each day. You'll be surprised how motivating it is. Some pedometers even show how many calories you are burning!

For many of you, these changes can easily be made on your own. But we know that for some of you these may seem like dramatic or even impossi-ble changes. Because of their importance in changing your gene-based risks, please don't hesitate to seek help from a professional, such as a regis-tered dietitian, licensed mental health professional, physician, or certified personal trainer.

STEP FOUR: FOLLOWING THE PHENOTYPE E DIET

The Phenotype E Diet helps you change from eating based on emotions to eating in response to hunger. It also turns your food-based weight gain triggers into weight loss triggers with a specific food list, structured meals, and sensible portions. As a result of the process, you will feel less deprived because you won't allow yourself to get ravenously hungry. You will also have more control over your emotions. This diet plan preempts reac-tionary behaviors on a cellular level and an emotional level with two sim-ple rules:

1. **Do not allow yourself to go more than two to three hours with-out eating.** Eating every two to three hours keeps your stress level down by consistently fueling the body and brain with the dietary chemicals needed to avoid glucose decreases and cortisol spurts. It raises your energy level by providing frequent healthy calories, and it satisfies your desire to eat.

2. **Eat a protein and a carbohydrate food at every mini-meal.** You can't eat just any food every two to three hours. You must eat the protein/carbohydrate combination to allay the constant urge to eat that stems

> The Phenotype E Diet combines protein and high fiber carbohydrate at each of your six minimeals.

The diet isn't totally inflexible. On some days, you may need to combine two minimeals to make a larger meal for dinner due to your schedule. As long as you don't go more than two to three hours without eating early in the day, you can combine the last two minimeals and have a larger dinner. For example, suppose you know you're going out to dinner with friends. The typical emotional eater would cut back on food early in the day to "save room" for the bigger meal at night. Don't do it! This sets you up to overeat. If you have your four minimeals during the day, you can safely eat a combined meal at night and not lose control.

from emotions. It will keep you feeling full and satisfied, because, taking longer to digest, it delays stomach emptying. Satiety refers to the process that determines the length of time between meals. Satiety value is greatest for protein, then fat, then carbohydrate. Fluids are less satiating than semisolids, which are less satiating than solids. Hot foods produce a greater feeling of satisfaction or satiety than cold foods. When you eat a protein/carb combo, glucose is released into the blood stream slowly rather than all at once, suppressing the insulin response, keeping blood sugar levels constant, and sustaining energy. Moreover, your emotions will be less volatile, not exacerbated by the intermittent hunger brought about by glucose fluctuations when you go without food or eat the wrong foods.

The Phenotype E Diet:

- Helps control your emotional eating with emotion-regulating foods so you can lose weight.
- Includes a minimeal every two to three hours to prevent emotional or stress eating.
- Includes a protein food and a carbohydrate food at every minimeal to produce satiety (fullness and satisfaction).
- Fights stress by increasing antioxidant intake from colorful fruits and vegetables.
- Adds calcium-rich foods to aid in weight loss.

Focus Foods

Research has demonstrated that specific foods will be critical to your success because the dietary chemicals they contain help dissipate emotions, stave off hunger, and/or optimize metabolism.

Omega-3 fatty acid–rich seafood: Fish is always a good low-calorie protein choice. Additionally, eating more fish may help stabilize Phenotype Es' moods. Global research studies in *The American Journal of Psychiatry* and *Psychopharmacology Update* concluded that the omega-3 fatty acids found in fish, eicosapentaenoic acid (EPA) and docosahexaenoic acid (DHA), seem to lessen depression. People with depression sometimes have too little EPA and DHA in their brain cell membranes. Correlating fish consumption and the rate of major depression country by country, studies have indicated that where fish consumption is the highest, the rates of depression are lowest. Fish such as mackerel, salmon, and tuna, in particular, are high in omega-3 fatty acids.

Scientists have established several means by which raising the concentration of these essential fatty acids in your blood will improve your mood. EPA and DHA accomplish higher production and utilization of serotonin and dopamine. They incorporate into brain cell membranes to facilitate cell signaling. The anti-inflammatory response that they produce benefits brain serotonin levels too.

Try to eat two to three omega-3 fatty acid–rich seafood choices each week. Choices of omega-3 seafood from highest to lowest are Pacific herring, Atlantic salmon, anchovies, Atlantic herring, Pacific mackerel, whitefish, Pacific sardines, oysters, Atlantic mackerel, bluefish, striped bass, albacore tuna, mussels, shrimp, snapper, and light tuna. Tuna comes in easy-to-use pouches that can be mixed with some chopped apple and a little light mayonnaise to make a great minimeal. If you're worried about mercury levels in seafood, Appendix H has a list of best choices.

Alpha-linolenic acid–rich foods: Canola oil, soybean oil, soybeans, wheat germ, ground flaxseed, and walnuts are abundant sources of the fatty acid alpha-linolenic acid (ALA). The human body converts ALA into DHA and EPA in modest amounts (about 5 to 15 percent). Since EPA and DHA are the important omega-3 fatty acids that soothe moods (as described

You can buy flaxseed already ground in many groceries and health food stores, or you can grind your own flaxseed in your coffee grinder. If it is ground, the body utilizes the ALA, lignans, and other healthy components, but if it is not ground, the flaxseed passes through the body as a fiber source only.

above), this is helpful, particularly for vegetarians, who don't get the benefit of seafood.

Calcium-rich dairy foods: The calcium in milk, yogurt, and cheese is every dieter's friend but is especially beneficial to Phenotype Es, who require the protein/carb mix to sustain positive emotions. Diets with little calcium stimulate fat-producing gene expression, what is called *lipogenesis.* High-calcium diets, by contrast, inhibit lipogenesis and accelerate *lipolysis,* which is the breakdown of stored fat. By increasing the metabolic rate (the rate at which calories are burned), they further reverse fat storage and prevent weight gain. Recent studies published in *The Journal of Nutrition* showed that in adults each 300 mg of calcium (for example, 1 cup of skim milk) was associated with an average of six pounds of weight loss. And among people consuming equal numbers of calories, people who consumed 1,000 mg of calcium from dairy foods daily lost more weight and fat than those consuming only 600 mg, the average intake for women in the United States.

Interestingly, data show that taking calcium in supplements does not necessarily lead to weight loss. The weight loss benefit of calcium-fortified foods such as juice, cereal, and bread hasn't yet been determined.

Eat dairy foods three times a day for a total of at least 1,000 mg. Dairy foods are also the perfect combination of protein and carbohydrate. Work them in as some of your allowed protein sources, using your hand as your portion-size tool (see Food List, page 193). They make an easy addition to your minimeals, with all of the prepackaged yogurt smoothies, cheese sticks, and flavored milks available in the grocery stores. Or try a latte with skim milk for your morning coffee.

Antioxidant-rich fruits and vegetables: Like pigments, fibers, and other plant constituents, antioxidants are among the large group of phytochemicals found naturally in foods that have a positive effect on health. Antioxidants such as beta-carotene and vitamin C are an important element for Phenotype Es because they reduce the effects of stress, which so often prompts emotional eating.

To explain how antioxidants optimize our health, we use a car analogy. Every day your car is exposed to air, humidity, and sometimes rain, snow, or even hail. If not protected, over a period of time the car will rust. Like rust, the unstable molecules called *free radicals* that result from stress and exposure to pollutants cause oxidization in living systems. Free radicals damage cells, disturb cells' ability to function normally, and deplete immunity. Like good detailing and a car cover, antioxidants act as a protective shield for cells, keeping them from the harmful effects of free radicals.

Colorful fruits and vegetables are the best sources of antioxidants. The brighter and more intense the produce's color, the more loaded it is with naturally occurring antioxidants. Some of the best sources of antioxidants are blueberries, cantaloupe, broccoli, spinach, asparagus, carrots, tomatoes, peaches, and sweet potatoes. To see more antioxidant sources, go to Appendix D.

FOCUS FOOD FREQUENCY

FOOD ITEM	FREQUENCY
Seafood	2–3 times per week
Walnuts	3 times per week
Wheat germ	3 times per week
Soybeans	Use as a meat substitute weekly
Canola/olive oil	Daily
Flaxseed meal	1 tablespoon 3 times per week
Calcium foods	3 times per day to equal 1,000–1,500 mg
Antioxidant foods	6–8 times daily

Begin with the Phenotype E *FAST TRACK* Two Weeks

With its quick results, the *FAST TRACK* Two Weeks get you motivated to keep going. The *FAST TRACK* is too severe for achieving long-term changes to your phenotype, but it will jump-start your weight loss. You'll begin to feel leaner, healthier and sexier within days. It uses the same Minimeal format as the Phenotype E Diets for men and women below, with the following exceptions:

1. Omit the number of proteins, carbohydrates and fats, as **bold-faced** in parentheses in the Minimeals below.
2. Omit the two fist-size 🍷 🍷 portions of "Sweets, Treats, and Alcohol" (see page 196) allowed each week.
3. Take a multivitamin/mineral supplement as well as the recommended additional vitamin C and vitamin E daily (see "Supplements" on page 205).
4. Start Week 3 with the full Phenotype E Diet.

THE PHENOTYPE E DIET FOR WOMEN

Select foods and portions for each minimeal from the Food List on page 193. Sample Menus using foods that fit the diet are on page 196.

Minimeal 1
1 Protein (any fist, ½ fist, or thumb[s] selection)
1 Carbohydrate
1 Fat
Freebie beverages

Minimeal 2
1 Protein (any fist, ½ fist, or thumb[s] selection)
1 Carbohydrate
Freebie beverages

Minimeal 3
2 Proteins (1 palm OR any 2: fist, ½ fist, or thumb[s] selections)
    (omit 1 protein for *FAST TRACK* Two Weeks)
1 Carbohydrate
Freebie vegetables
1 Fat
Freebie beverages

Minimeal 4
1 Protein (any fist, ½ fist, or thumb[s] selection)
1 Carbohydrate
Freebie vegetables
1 Fat **(omit for *FAST TRACK* Two Weeks)**
Freebie beverages

Minimeal 5
2 Proteins (1 palm OR any 2: fist, ½ fist, or thumb[s] selections)
    (omit 1 protein for *FAST TRACK* Two Weeks)
3 Carbohydrates **(omit 1 carbohydrate for *FAST TRACK* Two Weeks)**
Freebie Vegetables
1 Fat
Freebie beverages

(continued on next page)

Minimeal 6
1 Protein (any fist, ½ fist, or thumb[s] selection)
1 Carbohydrate
Freebie beverages

THE PHENOTYPE E DIET FOR MEN

Select your foods and portions for each minimeal from the Food List on page 193. Sample Menus using foods that fit the diet are on page 201.

Minimeal 1
1 Protein (any fist, ½ fist, or thumb[s] selection)
2 Carbohydrates
1 Fat
Freebie beverages

Minimeal 2
1 Protein (any fist, ½ fist, or thumb[s] selection)
1 Carbohydrate
1 Fat **(omit for *FAST TRACK* Two Weeks)**
Freebie beverages

Minimeal 3
2 Proteins (1 palm OR any 2: fist, ½ fist, or thumb[s] selections)
   (omit 1 protein for *FAST TRACK* Two Weeks)
3 Carbohydrates **(omit 1 carbohydrate for *FAST TRACK* Two Weeks)**
Freebie vegetables
1 Fat
Freebie beverages

Minimeal 4
1 Protein (any fist, ½ fist, or thumb[s] selection)
1 Carbohydrate
Freebie vegetables
1 Fat **(omit for *FAST TRACK* Two Weeks)**
Freebie beverages

Minimeal 5
2 Proteins (1 palm OR any 2: fist, ½ fist, or thumb[s] selections)
3 Carbohydrates **(omit 1 carbohydrate for *FAST TRACK* Two Weeks)**
Freebie Vegetables
1 Fat
Freebie beverages

Minimeal 6
1 Protein (any fist, ½ fist, or thumb[s] selection)
1 Carbohydrate
Freebie beverages

FOOD LIST

Very often "portion distortion" is a negative weight trigger, so reapportioning servings is a big part of triggering weight loss.

How much of each food should you eat? Use your hand as your guide. Eat the amount that you see; that is, the size of your fist, your palm, or your thumb. Focus Foods are in **bold type.**

 PALM

 FIST

 THUMB

Protein Sources

 Seafood. Poultry without skin, or lean cuts of meat such as loin, round, or cutlets of beef, pork, ham, veal, venison, lamb, etc.; cook by steaming, sautéing, broiling, or grilling. Meat alternative (**tofu, tempeh,** or other **soy product**)

Skim milk, buttermilk, evaporated skim milk, low-fat yogurt, low-fat cottage cheese, calcium-fortified soy milk, eggs such as Eggland's Best Eggs that are rich in omega-3 fatty acids (100 mg per egg), ricotta cheese (fat free)

½ Edamame, garbanzo, pinto, kidney, black, lima, or white beans; split, black-eyed, or field peas; lentils

Parmigiano-Reggiano, grana padana, string cheese, Neufchâtel (reduced-fat cream cheese), soy cheese, walnuts, peanut butter, almond butter or other nut butters, almonds, Brazil nuts, cashews, chestnuts, hazelnuts, macadamia nuts, mixed nuts, peanuts, pecans, pine nuts, pistachios, soy nuts, pumpkin seeds, sunflower seeds

Swiss, Cheddar, mozzarella, Romano, colby, feta, Gorgonzola, goat, or Monterey Jack cheese

Carbohydrate Sources

Whole grain bread, corn tortilla, whole wheat tortilla, whole grain English muffin or bagel, focaccia bread, whole wheat pita or ½ round whole grain lavash, whole grain crackers, corn bread, polenta, whole grain muffins, whole grain waffles or pancakes

Popped popcorn

High-fiber cereal, muesli

Apple, banana, berries, carambola (star fruit), cherries, citrus, grapes, kiwi fruit, melon, mango, nectarine, peach, pear, pineapple, plum

100% fruit juice, plain or calcium-fortified (limit to once a day)

> Check out the *Freebie* list for lots of veggies, including salad greens, tomatoes, carrots, etc., that you don't have to limit.

½ Grits; oatmeal; Wheatena; couscous; whole wheat pasta, pasta with at least 2 grams of fiber per serving; brown rice or other whole grain; garbanzo, pinto, kidney, black, lima, or white beans; split, black-eyed, or field peas; lentils; edamame; corn; green peas; potatoes with skin; acorn or butternut squash; sweet potatoes or yams; plantain

Dried fruit such as raisins, cherries, blueberries, apricots, plums, figs, etc.

Flaxseed meal, wheat germ

Fat Sources

MONOUNSATURATED FATS

Avocado, olives, hummus, almonds, Brazil nuts, cashews, chestnuts, hazelnuts, macadamia nuts, mixed nuts, peanuts, pecans, pine nuts, pistachios, **soy nuts, walnuts,** pumpkin seeds, safflower seeds, sesame seeds, sunflower seeds

Olive oil, canola oil, peanut oil, tahini paste, low-trans-fat margarines such as Olivio

POLYUNSATURATED FATS

Benecol Light or Take Control Light spread, salad dressing, light margarine, light mayonnaise, light salad dressing, low-trans-fat margarines such as Smart Balance

Benecol or Take Control spread, corn oil, safflower oil, soybean oil, sesame oil, sunflower oil, tartar sauce, salad dressing

Freebies

Beverages: Coffee, tea, diet soft drinks, club soda, carbonated or mineral water

Veggies: Artichoke, artichoke hearts, arugula, asparagus, bean sprouts, beets, Bibb lettuce, broccoli, Brussels sprouts, carrots, cauliflower, cabbage, celery, collard greens, cucumber, endive, eggplant, escarole, green beans, green onions or scallions, green, red, or yellow pepper, kale, kohlrabi, leeks, lettuce, mixed greens, mesclun, mushrooms, mustard greens, okra, onions, pea pods, radishes, romaine, spinach, summer squash, tomato, turnips, turnip greens, water chestnuts, zucchini

Miscellaneous: Broth or bouillon, ketchup, horseradish, lemon juice, lime juice, mustard, pickles, soy sauce, taco sauce, salsa, vinegars, garlic, fresh or dried herbs, pimento, spices, wine used in cooking, Worcestershire sauce, sugar substitutes

Sweets, Treats, and Alcohol

The Phenotype E Diet gives you two fists   of your choice per week to use as you desire.

Mimi, as an example, wrote, "One day Dad brought home a box of twenty-four Ding Dongs he was taking to one of the businesses. It sat on the counter for two days.

> To use the two fists 🖐 🖐 as treats, you don't have to subtract anything from the Phenotype E Diet. These treats are already calculated into your diet.

Finally I couldn't stand it anymore, grabbed one, and took a bite. I felt like I was dipping snuff, but I just had to taste the chocolate. Now I realize that I really can't have foods like this around because I can't stop thinking about them. I have to tell you, what has really helped me is that I don't feel deprived since I can have the two fists of treats during the week as part of my diet. On Valentine's Day, I used them all in one day."

> If certain foods trigger you to overeat, stay away from them. Don't tempt yourself by keeping them at home or at work. Make them difficult to get and difficult to eat. Many of our clients keep treats at home for their children, but they make it a point to choose treats that won't tempt them. One client bought gummi worms for her children because those definitely were not high on her list of appealing foods.

SAMPLE MENUS

On days when you're rushed, use the NO-TIME Menus. MORE-TIME Menus are for days when you can cook leisurely. The menus are also meant to serve as a guide for eating out.

NO-TIME Menu E for Women

MINIMEAL 1

 Toasted almond muesli sprinkled with:

 Golden raisins and flaxseed meal combined

Skim milk/low-fat soy milk

Freebie beverages

MINIMEAL 2

  Laughing Cow cheese (light)

 Triscuits (low-fat version)

Freebie beverages

Laughing Cow cheese doesn't require refrigeration. Look for it in a round cardboard container with a smiling cow on the label.

MINIMEAL 3

 Whole wheat pita pocket stuffed with:

> *Freebie* Sliced bright red or green bell peppers

> *Freebie* Cucumber rounds

> *Freebie* Fresh baby spinach leaves

 Red sockeye salmon (canned) mixed with:

> Cashews, chopped

> Mayonnaise (light)

Freebie vegetables

Freebie beverages

MINIMEAL 4

 Cappuccino soy milk

 Whole grain lavash (flat bread) **or** whole wheat pita with

>   hummus

Freebie vegetables

Freebie beverages

MINIMEAL 5

Veggie and cheese pizza (ask for extra veggies)

Freebie Mixed salad greens topped with:

> Granny Smith apple, sliced

> Raspberry walnut vinaigrette (light, such as Ken's)

Freebie vegetables

Freebie beverages

MINIMEAL 6

Chocolate yogurt (such as Stonyfield's organic) topped with:

> Fresh sliced strawberries

Freebie beverages

MORE-TIME Menu E for Women

MINIMEAL 1

½ Irish steel-cut oatmeal such as McCann's prepared with

> low-fat soy milk/skim milk

Be sure to check the product label. Not all soy milk is low fat.

Top with:

> ½ Fresh raspberries

> Walnuts

Freebie Green tea or coffee

MINIMEAL 2

 Goat cheese with herbs

 Rosemary focaccia bread

Freebie beverages

MINIMEAL 3

South of the Border Salad

      Freebie Spring mix salad greens

        Grilled spicy chicken strips

SLATER'S MEXICAN FIESTA RUB

2 teaspoons chili powder
2 teaspoons garlic powder
2 teaspoons onion powder
2 teaspoons cumin
½ teaspoon black pepper
½ teaspoon oregano
Splash of balsamic vinegar

Mix dry ingredients and whisk in vinegar to form a thick paste. Rub paste over chicken before grilling.

  ½  Yellow corn

  ½ Black beans

Freebie Diced tomatoes and onions

  Thousand Island dressing (light)

Freebie beverages

MINIMEAL 4

 Polenta with pine nuts and Parmigiano-Reggiano cheese

> Wedge of polenta topped with:

> Parmigiano-Reggiano cheese

> *Freebie* Diced tomatoes

> Pine nuts

Freebie vegetables

Freebie beverages

MINIMEAL 5

 Mussels with fresh-squeezed lemon juice and garlic

 Spicy sweet potato wedges

SPICY SWEET POTATO WEDGES

Slice potato into thick wedges and put into a zip-top bag along with spicy seasoning such as Emeril's. Shake and bake at 400 degrees for 20–25 minutes.

 So Easy Caesar Salad (see NO-TIME Recipes in Appendix C)

 Golden pineapple chunks with fresh strawberries

Freebie vegetables

Freebie beverages

MINIMEAL 6

 French vanilla low-fat yogurt topped with:

 Fresh peach, sliced

Freebie beverages

NO-TIME Menu E for Men

MINIMEAL 1

  Toasted almond muesli with:

 Golden raisins

 Ground flaxseed meal

 Skim milk/low-fat soy milk

Freebie beverages

> You can buy flaxseed already ground in many groceries and health food stores, or you can grind your own flaxseed in your coffee grinder. If it is ground, the body utilizes the ALA, lignans, and other healthy components, but if it is not ground, the flaxseed passes through the body as a fiber source only.

MINIMEAL 2

  Laughing Cow cheese (light)

 Triscuits (low-fat version)

Freebie beverages

> Laughing Cow cheese doesn't require refrigeration. Look for it in a round cardboard container with a smiling cow on the label.

MINIMEAL 3

 Whole wheat pita pocket stuffed with:

Freebie Sliced bright red or green bell peppers (can also be eaten on the side with balsamic vinegar)

Freebie Cucumber rounds (can also be eaten on the side)

Freebie Fresh baby spinach leaves

Red sockeye salmon (canned) mixed with:

> Cashews, chopped

> Mayonnaise (light)

Freebie vegetables

 Blueberry fruit smoothie:

> ½ Skim milk/low fat vanilla soymilk

> ½ Frozen blueberries

Place in blender and blend for 30–60 seconds.

Freebie beverages

MINIMEAL 4

1 Odwalla Bar: Chocolate

or

1 Powerbar Harvest: Peanut Butter Chocolate Chip (see Appendix A for tips on finding the best bars)

Freebie beverages

MINIMEAL 5

 Veggie and cheese pizza (ask for extra veggies)

Freebie Mixed salad greens topped with:

> Granny Smith apple, sliced

>   Raspberry walnut vinaigrette (light, such as Ken's)

Freebie vegetables

Freebie beverages

MINIMEAL 6

  Mozzarella string cheese

 Fresh sliced strawberries

Freebie beverages

MORE-TIME Menu E for Men

MINIMEAL 1

 Irish steel-cut oatmeal such as McCann's prepared with

 low-fat soy milk/skim milk

Be sure to check the product label. Not all soy milk is low fat.

Top with:

½ Fresh raspberries

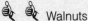 Walnuts

Freebie Green tea or coffee

MINIMEAL 2

  Rosemary focaccia bread

 Goat cheese with herbs

Freebie beverages

MINIMEAL 3

 Whole wheat or corn tortilla stuffed with:

  Grilled spicy chicken strips

 Shredded Mexican cheese blend

Freebie Chunky salsa

SLATER'S MEXICAN FIESTA RUB

2 teaspoons chili powder
2 teaspoons garlic powder
2 teaspoons onion powder
2 teaspoons cumin
½ teaspoon black pepper
½ teaspoon oregano
Splash of balsamic vinegar

Mix dry ingredients and whisk in vinegar to form a thick paste. Rub paste over chicken before grilling.

Southwest Salad

> *Freebie* Spring mix salad greens
>
> ½ Yellow corn
>
> ½ Black beans
>
> *Freebie* Diced tomatoes and onions
>
>   Thousand Island dressing (light)

 Kiwi fruit

Freebie vegetables

Freebie beverages

MINIMEAL 4

 Polenta with pine nuts and Parmigiano-Reggiano cheese

Wedge of polenta topped with:

> *Freebie* Diced tomatoes
>
> Pine nuts

Parmigiano-Reggiano cheese

Freebie vegetables

Freebie beverages

MINIMEAL 5

  Mussels with fresh-squeezed lemon juice and garlic

 Spicy sweet potato wedges

 So Easy Caesar Salad (see NO-TIME Recipes in Appendix C)

 Golden pineapple chunks with fresh strawberries

Freebie beverages and vegetables

SPICY SWEET POTATO WEDGES

Slice potato into thick wedges and put into a zip-top bag along with spicy seasoning such as Emeril's. Shake and bake at 400 degrees for 20–25 minutes.

MINIMEAL 6

 French vanilla low-fat yogurt topped with:

 Fresh peach, sliced

Freebie beverages

Supplements

St. John's wort (Hypericum perforatum): One of the most popular herbal remedies in the United States, St. John's wort is used to treat mild depression and anxiety. It is hence a natural choice for Phenotype Es. However, if you presently take St. John's wort or are considering it, we have several caveats. Few people can accurately judge whether their depression is mild, moderate, or severe. If you are feeling depressed, before you try to self-medicate, it's important to see your physician or a licensed mental health professional for an assessment and recommendations. The most successful treatment for depression is usually a combination of talk therapy and medication. Neither works as well alone. If your depression is diagnosed as being in the mild category, ask about trying St. John's wort.

Purchase a St. John's wort supplement with its active compounds, the reddish pigment hypericin, and flavonoids from the flowers and leaves. Do not mix St. John's wort with prescription medications unless approved by your physician, because St. John's wort activates liver enzymes that metabolize drugs. Also, St. John's wort may reduce the effectiveness of medications such as protease inhibitors, cyclosporine, digoxin, warfarin, chemotherapy drugs, antipsychotics, cholesterol-lowering agents, and theophylline. If you are already taking antidepressants such as monoamine oxidase inhibitors (MAOIs), selective serotonin reuptake inhibitors (SSRIs), other antidepressants, SAMe, or antimigraine medications, you should not take St. John's wort.

St. John's wort can also interfere with the absorption of iron and other minerals. In some cases it has caused breakthrough bleeding in women and rendered the birth control pill less effective. It's also important to note that St. John's wort can prolong the side effects of anesthesia, so be sure to let your doctor and anesthesiologist know about any supplements you are taking prior to surgery. Side effects may occasionally include fatigue, allergic skin reactions, headaches, or gastrointestinal complaints.

S-Adenosyl-L-methionine (SAMe): This molecule occurs naturally in the body and is produced by a reaction between the amino acid methionine, and adenosine triphosphate (ATP), a compound used by cells to perform all types of tasks. SAMe is involved in the production of the neurotransmitters (brain chemicals) serotonin, dopamine, and melatonin, which influence mood, and the components of cartilage, which support bone structure and strength. As a supplement, it is used for its antidepressant benefits and for osteoarthritis.

The cautionary note for St. John's wort applies to SAMe too. Before you try to self-medicate, discuss your condition and SAMe with your physician or a licensed mental health professional. As with St. John's wort, SAMe should not be combined with prescription antidepressants such as tricyclic antidepressants (TCAs), selective serotonin reuptake inhibitors (SSRIs), nor with monoamine oxidase inhibitors (MAOIs). If SAMe is taken, St. John's wort should not be used. Individuals with bipolar (manic-depressive) disorder should be aware that SAMe can trigger a manic phase.

Last, do not use SAMe if you are nursing or pregnant. Also, SAMe may be contraindicated for cardiac patients, since it can elevate homocysteine levels in the blood, a risk factor for heart disease. It may lower blood digoxin levels by up to 25 percent, so it is not recommended for cardiac patients who are using digoxin to strengthen their heart muscle contractions.

Omega-3 fatty acids: Omega-3 fats include eicosapentaenoic acid (EPA) and docosahexaenoic acid (DHA), and are common in the oils of fish. As mentioned in Focus Foods, they can also be made within your body from a precursor substance called alpha-linolenic acid (ALA) found in plant foods such as walnuts and flaxseed meals. Food sources of omega-3 fatty acids and ALA foods are included in your Focus Foods list. If you do not eat fish, fish oil supplements containing omega-3 fatty acids have been shown to have similar mood-stabilizing properties, triglyceride- and blood pressure–lowering effects, and anti-inflammatory effects, such as helping to prevent relapse in Crohn's disease or rheumatoid arthritis.

If you are hemophiliac, taking prescription blood thinners such as warfarin (Coumadin) or heparin, or expecting to undergo surgery, fish oil supplements should be used only under a physician's care.

5-HTP: 5-hydroxytryptophan (5-HTP) is used as a supplement for depression and for insomnia. Since the body uses 5-HTP to make serotonin, providing it by taking a supplement can raise brain serotonin levels. According to a study in the journal *Psychopathology,* 5-HTP was compared as a treatment for depression with an antidepressant in the SSRI family (fluvoxamine). In this study, both were effective in treating depression, but 5-HTP users reported fewer and less severe side effects. Because 5-HTP raises serotonin levels like St. John's wort and SAMe, do not use it if you are taking other antidepressant medications such as MAOI, SSRIs, or serotonin receptor agonists.

Valerian (*Valeriana officinalis*): Insomnia can be a problem for Phenotype Es. Valerian, an age-old folk treatment for sleeplessness, is an accepted sleep aid and is most useful when taken over time for chronic sleep problems. Its mechanism of action is not well understood, but it may affect the brain's production of gamma-aminobutyric acid (GABA), a chemical associated with reducing anxiety. Studies have shown that it may take two to four weeks of regular use to produce significantly improved sleep. So if your sleeping problem is situational and lasts for a short time, for example after a stressful incident that disrupts sleep for a night or two, valerian may not be much help. *It should not be used in addition to other medications for insomnia or anti-anxiety medications, such as benzodiazapenes (Ativan or Xanax).*

SUPPLEMENT RECOMMENDATIONS AND DOSES

SUPPLEMENT	DOSE
Multivitamin/mineral	Daily
Vitamin C	250 mg daily

(continued on next page)

SUPPLEMENT	DOSE
Vitamin E	200 IU mixed tocopherols for women daily; 400 IU mixed tocopherols for men daily
St. John's wort	900 mg per day in three divided doses of 300 mg each to provide 0.2–1 mg of total hypericin or 2–4.5% hyperforin. Take for 4–6 weeks and then evaluate for improvement. Do not take if you are using valerian or SAMe.
SAMe	400 to 800 mg is the generally recommended daily dose. Start with a dose of 200 mg of SAMe twice a day. Continue that dose for two weeks. If no improvement, increase dosage to 200 mg three to four times a day. When improvement in mood has been achieved, you can try gradually reducing the dose. 200 mg twice a day appears to be the minimum effective maintenance dose. If SAMe is taken, St. John's wort should not be used.
5-HTP	100–300 mg three times daily
Omega-3 or fish oil supplements	Take one 1,000 mg capsule three times per day with meals; this is equivalent to approximately 900 mg per day total of EPA and DHA, since most 1,000 mg capsules contain 180 mg EPA and 120 mg DHA each
Valerian	1,000 mg of dried valerian root in tablet form taken 30–60 minutes before bedtime

The Diet You Can't Blow

No one, not even nutritionists, eats perfectly all the time. If you run into an occasional snag where you get off track for some reason—maybe it's the holidays or vacation time—don't be discouraged. Sometimes it's the circumstances, sometimes it's the people you're with, sometimes it's just not convenient to eat the right thing, and sometimes you just want a treat.

When food lover Nick first attempted the Phenotype E Diet, he'd occasionally blow his diet by drinking too much wine with his friends. He'd tell himself he had failed and feel there was no point in continuing. Phenotype Es and feelings of failure go hand in hand. High emotions provide the rationale for reverting to overeating. But change is a process, and any number of temptations can intervene. Setbacks happen.

Pinpoint what triggered the setback, learn from it, regain your confidence, and go on from there. One trick is to look ahead and plan ahead to deal with setbacks, which often occur during emotionally charged holidays. Decide when you want to use your two fists of treats, as Tamara does. "When I don't succeed," wrote Tamara, "I let myself down. But I've learned there will be setbacks and to not expect myself to be perfect—nobody is. I just try to get back on track the next day. One trick I've mastered for holidays and parties is to fill my glass with diet 7 UP and about one ounce of wine—then I have my spritzer without all the calories and still feel a part of the festivities."

If you find that you have regained a little weight, you can go back to the *FAST TRACK* Two Weeks and then to the Phenotype E Diet until you drop the extra pounds. When you do, continue on with the Phenotype E Maintenance Diet. Like Nick, you'll begin to understand that just because you don't always follow the diet perfectly doesn't mean you aren't progressing. Remember that conquering emotional eating is not so much about weight loss as it is about coming to grips with emotional ups and downs.

Stopped losing weight? Refer to the "How to Deal with Plateaus" on page 28 and reboot your diet with another *FAST TRACK* Two Weeks.

The Phenotype E Maintenance Diet

Remember when you started on the Phenotype E Diet? In a few days, something inside just seemed to click and you began to lose weight, feel better, and feel healthier. That will not change. When you reach your goal weight, you are ready to move on to the Phenotype E Maintenance Diet.

The diet has the same backbone Focus Foods, so it will keep you satisfied and your weight constant along with regular physical activity.

THE PHENOTYPE E
MAINTENANCE DIET FOR WOMEN

Minimeal 1
1 Protein (any fist, ½ fist, or thumb[s] selection)
2 Carbohydrates
1 Fat
Freebie beverages

Minimeal 2
1 Protein (any fist, ½ fist, or thumb[s] selection)
1 Carbohydrate
Freebie beverages

Minimeal 3
2 Proteins (1 palm OR any 2: fist, ½ fist, or thumb[s] selections)
2 Carbohydrates
Freebie vegetables
1 Fat
Freebie beverages

Minimeal 4
1 Protein (any fist, ½ fist, or thumb[s] selection)
1 Carbohydrate
Freebie vegetables
1 Fat
Freebie beverages

Minimeal 5
2 Proteins (1 palm OR any 2: fist, ½ fist, or thumb[s] selections)
3 Carbohydrates
Freebie Vegetables
2 Fats
Freebie beverages

Minimeal 6
1 Protein (any fist, ½ fist, or thumb[s] selection)
1 Carbohydrate
Freebie beverages

THE PHENOTYPE E
MAINTENANCE DIET FOR MEN

Minimeal 1
1 Protein (any fist, ½ fist, or thumb[s] selection)
2 Carbohydrates
1 Fat
Freebie beverages

Minimeal 2
1 Protein (any fist, ½ fist, or thumb[s] selection)
1 Carbohydrate
1 Fat
Freebie beverages

Minimeal 3
2 Proteins (1 palm OR any 2: fist, ½ fist, or thumb[s] selections)
3 Carbohydrates
Freebie vegetables
1 Fat
Freebie beverages

Minimeal 4
1 Protein (any fist, ½ fist, or thumb[s] selection)
2 Carbohydrates
Freebie vegetables
1 Fat
Freebie beverages

Minimeal 5
2 Proteins (1 palm OR any 2: fist, ½ fist, or thumb[s] selections)
3 Carbohydrates
Freebie vegetables
2 Fats
Freebie beverages

Minimeal 6
1 Protein (any fist, ½ fist, or thumb[s] selection)
1 Carbohydrate
Freebie beverages

CHAPTER 9

The Phenotype H Diet

Outsmarting Hormone–
Linked Weight Gain

Melissa's Story

"I've always had 'female problems.' My mother did, too."

"As far back as I can remember, I've had terrible cravings the week before my period, and I would eat nonstop. I mean, I still do. I usually start with a Coke during my early-afternoon slump to keep me going. After a microwave dinner, I move on to a bag of chocolate brownie bites, but I don't stop there, I take Ben & Jerry's to bed with me. Chubby Hubby is my favorite, but it's not my hubby who's chubby; it's me! And I haven't even mentioned my mood swings. My mood swings make me horrible to be around. I can hardly stand myself at times."

Once a tall, curvaceous blonde, Melissa had become what she described as "big, blond, and bloated" when she entered our PMS seminar. Like many women, Melissa's weight started the uphill climb when she hit her 30s. Before that, weight gain really wasn't an issue. She ate when she felt like it; she played tennis three or four times a week and water-skied nearly every weekend. She was young, active, and could eat her way through cravings and mood swings without gaining a single pound. But at age 41, it's a different story. As an emergency room nurse for the last eight years, she was skilled, knowledgeable, and worked with grace under intense pressure. Her hectic schedule provided little room for real meals. So Melissa ate sporadically out of vending machines and stashed chocolate in her locker, telling herself it was for the week before her period. But the chocolate never lasted that long. Whenever she was hungry, she munched on it, sometimes all month long. This led to a ten-pound gain she could never seem to lose.

"I just can't control myself. I go on and off diets every single month. I'm on for two weeks and then off for two weeks—the week before and during my period. How can I possibly lose any weight? Any pounds I may have lost, I put right back on during my monthly eat-a-thon."

Melissa is a classic PMS eater. Her weight fate is tied to eating habits resulting from her monthly hormonal swings.

Samantha's Story

"I gained fifty pounds with my daughter, lost twenty, and then gained another fifty pounds with my son."

Imagine the perfect early-summer wedding. It's unseasonably cool, with a warm breeze blowing. A petite 5'5", 125-pound bride carries a bouquet of fragrant, dewy gardenias that lightly scent the air as she strolls down the aisle. Samantha can still picture it as if it were yesterday. It was her dream come true and she was a vision of loveliness, happiness, and health. Only five years later, weighing 205 pounds after the birth of her second child, Samantha hated to look in the mirror. During her pregnancies she'd developed poor eating habits, and stress worsened them after her children were born. Samantha had become the proverbial thin wife trapped inside a postpartum body.

"During the six months after my son was born, I lost forty pounds through starving and skipping meals. I was still at least forty pounds overweight and exhausted all the time, with no energy. Really, who has time to eat properly with two children under the age of two? Most nights we grabbed fast food or wings on the way home from day care and only ate together as a family on weekends, when I might have time to cook.

"I'd had enough! I made up my mind to get some help. Keeping the hormonal cravings log seemed like one more thing to do. But it sure showed me how chaotic and totally unplanned my eating had become. Following the Phenotype H Diet has been easier than I expected, especially the NO-TIME Menus (which I'm sure were designed just for me). I'm steadily losing weight without starving, and I'm no longer the sporadic eater that I once was."

Paula's Story

"My girlfriends and I call this bulge the 'menopot.' I feel like I have to work harder than ever just to maintain, much less to lose, weight."

What if you were a dietitian, knew what to eat, had always been slim, and then menopause hit? Our colleague Paula explained it like this: "I never had a weight problem until menopause. Now I have this roll under my bra strap and around my stomach that I never had before. The hot flashes, night sweats, and mood swings make me feel like I'm on a roller coaster that I can't get off, and cravings are driving me crazy. My eating has become so sporadic—all based on my hormone ups and downs. What really bugs me is that I think I'm eating about the same amount of calories and exercising like I always have, but I keep gaining weight where I don't want it.

"The real kicker was when the cashier at the grocery said to me, 'You must be so excited, when is your baby due?' I guess it was nice that she thought I was young enough to have a baby, but even if I may look like I'm four months pregnant, <u>I'm certainly not.</u> Is it all downhill from here?"

Midlife hormone changes had thrown Paula for a loop. She needed to rethink her eating and lifestyle to overcome this hormonal phase.

If you are overweight and a Phenotype H, you answered "yes" to some of these statements in the Phenotype Assessment:

- I have gained more than the recommended weight gain for pregnancy and kept it on.
- My eating increases or changes significantly with my menstrual cycle.
- I experience food cravings during the two weeks before my period.
- I am experiencing hot flashes, mood swings, and night sweats.
- I had a pear-shaped body at one time but now have an apple-shaped body.
- I have gained 10 pounds or more excess weight with menopause.

STEP ONE: UNDERSTANDING YOUR PHENOTYPE

Phenotype Hs gain weight in association with a genetic tendency for female hormone fluctuations. Perhaps you overeat during the week before your period. Maybe you gained too much weight during pregnancy and have been unable to lose it. Or has menopause given you a "menopot"? If any of these conditions describes you, this is your phenotype. Research establishes a strong connection between weight gain and hormone variability. Interdependent, both stem from a common genetic grouping that we call Phenotype H.

The prevalence of obesity in women has doubled in the last twenty years.

Hormone levels fluctuate during critical, genetically programmed intervals in a woman's life—premenstrually and during pregnancy and menopause. The fluctuations increase the risk for becoming overweight, primarily because they provoke sporadic overeating. These events are hormonally and, in some cases, genetically induced. In all three cases, women inherit the genes, but their lifestyle, their eating habits, and behavior have as much to do with their weight as their genes do.

On the following pages, have a look at whatever section most describes your problem: "Weight Gain and PMS," "Weight Gain from Pregnancy," or "Weight Gain and Menopause." Then go to the Food Record section on page 222.

SAY GOOD-BYE TO HORMONAL BLOAT

When you look in the mirror, do you see a swollen version of yourself? Intermittent spikes in progesterone that occur throughout a woman's life increase her desire for salt that leads to water retention. Regardless of which critical hormonal stage you are in, changes in your tried-and-true habits can diminish the fluid retention and the puffiness. These include:

- Drinking plenty of water
- Working up a sweat with regular exercise
- Cutting back on your salt and sodium intake
- Eating more diuretic foods

These methods, reviewed in more detail in Focus Foods, help maintain the body's delicate balance of electrolytes (sodium, potassium, chloride) by flushing out the excess through urination and thus alleviating some of that "swollen" feeling.

Weight Gain and PMS

Premenstrual syndrome (PMS) includes a number of emotional and physical symptoms that occur a week to ten days prior to the beginning of your period, correlating to the monthly ebb and rise of various hormones. Twenty to 50 percent of women report experiencing PMS. That's a lot of women dealing with hormone-related issues, who often find their comfort in food.

A study reported in *Psychological Medicine* estimated that PMS is inherited in about 30 to 40 percent of all cases. Likewise, a study published in *Obstetrics and Gynecology* reported PMS symptoms in mothers' coinciding with an increased predisposition to PMS in their daughters. Data from twin studies also supports the issue of inherited risk. Another study reported in *The British Journal of Psychiatry* concluded that identical twins were twice as likely as fraternal twins to have similar PMS symptom severity scores. What this means is that your genes probably delivered you to Phenotype H, and likely your eating habits and behavior are opening and activating this genetic package.

Probably PMS, to some degree, first manifested when you were a teen. Puberty conveys dramatic changes to young women's bodies, as a means of preparing for potential childbearing, which will require wider hips, developed breasts, and the associated muscle and fat tissue. Hormonal signals—transported by estrogen, progesterone, testosterone, and other hormones—drive women to consume more calories, particularly during the *luteal phase,* the two weeks prior to the menstrual period. Estrogen and serotonin levels decline during these two weeks and progesterone spikes, setting off internal alarms that make women long for extra calories—and extra calories of a specific nature that we'll explain further. Healthy women

HOW CAN YOU TELL IF YOU HAVE PMS?

Five or more of the following symptoms must occur during the week to 10 days prior to the menstrual period for most cycles: moodiness, irritability, fatigue, inability to sleep, feeling out of control, increased food intake, cravings, headaches, weight gain, and bloating. At least one symptom must be moodiness or irritability. In order to meet the more extreme diagnosis of premenstrual dysphoric disorder (PDD), the symptoms must be debilitating enough to interfere with everyday work and social activities or relationships.

typically consume between 90 and 500 calories per day more premenstrually, but overeating can result in too much weight gain.

Serotonin is the neurotransmitter that gives you a feeling of calmness, decreased anxiety, and improved mood. Decreased levels of serotonin brought about during the luteal phase make women more sensitive and prone to irritability. Because food contains dietary chemicals that stimulate a series of actions that can affect serotonin levels, it is not illogical that women eat to overcome their PMS mood swings. The problem is that many of the foods they eat, while they do have a temporary effect, do not sustain their feelings of well-being. And if they do not work the calories off by exercising, these foods also lead to weight gain.

Interestingly, premenstrual food cravings center not on protein but on foods high in sugar, fat, and salt. Each of these cravings ties to premenstrual body chemistry: sugar and fat to the diminishing serotonin levels and salt to lower sodium levels.

When you eat carbohydrate—especially a refined carbohydrate such as sugar—your blood glucose levels rise and trigger the release of insulin. Insulin causes the large neutral amino acids (LNAAs)—tyrosine, phenylalanine, leucine, and isoleucine—to be taken up into muscle. At the same time, another LNAA, tryptophan, competes with these other LNAAs for the same transport molecule to get into the brain. Consuming a meal of pure carbohydrate increases the ratio of tryptophan to these other LNAAs in the blood. Hence, more tryptophan makes its way to the brain, where it converts to serotonin. That's why women reach for refined sugars and carbohydrates as part of their PMS, because the serotonin it produces contributes to making them feel better. The problem is that the "high" is brief.

High-fat foods deliver their own "feel-good" response by releasing endorphins, the same mood-enhancing neurochemicals released during exercise. Endorphins are morphinelike chemicals that exert analgesic effects by binding to opiate receptors on brain cells and increasing the pain threshold.

When the hormone progesterone rises abruptly, as it does once a month, its action as a diuretic causes women to excrete sodium. They then reach for more sodium, usually as salt on high-fat foods such as chips and fries.

What is the most frequently reported craving in women during PMS? You guessed it, *chocolate*. In a study of college students published in *Appetite,* the number of women who craved chocolate was 25 percent higher than in men. Because of its sugar content, chocolate can increase brain serotonin levels and, due to its fat content, in-

> For PMS, try lowering your sodium intake as much as possible during the week to ten days prior to your period. See Focus Foods for how-to recommendations.

Dying for chocolate? Satisfy the urge with your two fistfuls of "Sweets, Treats, and Alcohol" bonus during part of each week of your Phenotype H Diet.

crease endorphins at the same time. This combination of brain chemicals is often described as "optimal brain happiness."

A diet high in carbohydrate helps improve moods and the sense of well-being during the premenstrual seven to ten days. Some types of protein have a better effect on mood and on menstrual pain than others; we've highlighted these in the Focus Foods section.

Women with PMS also drink more caffeine-containing beverages than women without PMS. Unfortunately, consuming caffeine during the luteal phase may be counterproductive. Drinking approximately 5 cups or more of caffeine-containing beverages daily was associated with significant increases in both the prevalence and severity of PMS symptoms, according to a study published in the *American Journal of Public Health*. Decreasing or eliminating caffeine consumption during the two weeks prior to menstrual flow may reduce symptoms. In a later study of Chinese women published in the same journal, 4½ to 8 cups of tea was also linked to increasing prevalence of PMS symptoms. Researchers postulate that the caffeine in the tea was the contributing factor. Look on the following page for the caffeine content in various beverages.

Typical PMS food choices can deprive your body of beneficial minerals because the craved foods aren't necessarily healthy. As an example, we suggested that Melissa supplement her diet with calcium-rich foods during the two weeks prior to her period. As a routine, this helps relieve her symptoms and gives her better control over her cravings and thus her food selections. The result? She's taken off those extra ten pounds, and they've stayed off.

During the luteal phases, the basal metabolic rate (the rate at which calories burn while you are at rest) speeds up while you are asleep, burning extra calories. This contributes to the PMS-stimulated appetite, again signaling women to consume additional calories. The problem is that without exercise, daytime metabolism remains constant and many Phenotype Hs may not use as many calories as they are consuming. Prior generations were more active. Our sedentary lifestyle does nothing to mitigate the effects of PMS, because they deprive women's bodies of the hormone-balancing *and calorie-burning* effects of exercise. You will read more about this in Step Three.

If your weight gain is associated with PMS and not with pregnancy or menopause, you're ready to move on to Step Two on page 222.

CAFFEINE CONTENT IN VARIOUS BEVERAGES

BEVERAGE	SERVING SIZE	CAFFEINE IN MILLIGRAMS	
		AVERAGE	RANGE
Canned iced tea	1 cup (8 oz.)	17	10–24
Chocolate milk	1 cup (8 oz.)	5	2–7
Coffee, drip	1 cup (8 oz.)	184	176–240
Coffee, instant	1 cup (8 oz.)	104	65–120
Coffee, decaf	1 cup (8 oz.)	5	3–8
Coffee, espresso	¼ cup (2 oz.)	100	80–120
Cola soft drink	1 cup (8 oz.)	30	29–39
Hot chocolate	1 cup (8 oz.)	6	3–32
Tea, brewed, U.S. brand	1 cup (8 oz.)	47	32–144
Tea, brewed, imported	1 cup (8 oz.)	60	40–176
Tea, green	1 cup (8 oz.)	15	10–25
Tea, instant	1 cup (8 oz.)	30	20–50

Weight Gain from Pregnancy

A weight gain of at least 11 pounds occurs most commonly between ages 25 and 34 and affects twice as many women as men, largely as a result of the weight women gain during pregnancy, according to the evidence. Women keep or gain weight following pregnancy for a variety of reasons. For a start, they may have put on too many pounds during pregnancy; pounds not required for the fetus' development may be difficult to lose. They may also have trouble reining in the larger appetite they cultivated during pregnancy. A more stressful lifestyle such as Samantha's also works against weight loss because women need to plan for better food choices and exercise and may not take the time to do so. Postpartum and ongoing depression can lead to weight gain, too. Finally, although the jury is still out on whether women inherit a genetic tendency to weight gain after pregnancy, it is apparent that they often inherit habits—such as eating preferences and sedentary behaviors—that send extra weight to their hips and buttocks. Yet as our own clients and patients have demonstrated, these habits can change.

The average weight gain during pregnancy is 25 to 35 pounds, and this requires only 200 extra calories a day for most women. In a study reported in the *Journal of the American Dietetic Association,* only 38 percent gained the recommended amount of weight during pregnancy. Of the other 62 percent, many gained substantially more, and some gained less.

A study of 274 women reported in *Obstetrics and Gynecology* found that those with the highest rates of pregnancy weight gain had more body fat and a higher *body mass index* (BMI) at both six weeks and six months post-partum. (BMI is a measure of body fatness based on height and weight.) The excess weight gained didn't enhance the baby's growth; it enhanced the mother's rear end!

Another study, reported in the *American Journal of Public Health,* found that 34 percent of women with a high BMI who gained more than 25 pounds during pregnancy retained more than 14 pounds several months after delivery. Clearly, the hormone-intense interval of pregnancy and postpartum is a high-risk time for weight gain. Research reported in *The Lancet* found that for women who delay pregnancy until later in life, the risk of excess weight gain increases.

Typically, the greatest amount of weight lost after pregnancy occurs in the first three months and then proceeds slowly and steadily until six months, after which the weight loss decreases significantly or ends. This is because hormones take about six months to renormalize, whether women are overweight or not. The average pregnancy appetite needs to readjust to around 1,800 calories per day, which can be tough to accomplish. Unfortunately, many women have trouble losing the appetite they've cultivated for the last nine months.

A University of Greenwich study led by Dr. Helen Hunt found that increased food intake, not lack of exercise, was the main reason for continued weight gain after delivery. More than a fifth of women studied admitted that they were eating more after they gave birth than before. This could be because they were more likely to be at home, where food was more accessible. Dr. Hunt's researchers also found data suggesting that women with overweight mothers gain weight, possibly for genetic reasons; however the pattern did not trace to fathers. Therefore, the tendency may also be due to similar lifestyles—similar food choices and behaviors, and so on—as we mentioned earlier.

Depression during pregnancy and postpartum depression may play a role in weight gain and weight retention. A recent study reported in the *Journal of Women's Health* found that 20 percent of women meet the criteria for depression while pregnant and 86 percent of those received no treatment. From research and from clients' experience, we know that foods affect depression. A National Institute of Health study, as an example, focused on mothers who ate fish beginning after the first eight weeks of pregnancy and continued until eight months postpartum. Those who ate no seafood had nearly twice the rate of depression as those who ate ten ounces of fish daily. That's a lot of fish, but the relationship between the fish and depression is the important part: the more omega-3 fatty acids were consumed in fish, the lower the risk of depression. The Phenotype H Diet Focus Foods (a list of foods chosen specifically for this phenotype) include fish and other food sources of omega-3 fatty acids.

Nursing, in addition to providing the ideal fast food for your baby, may give you a head start on losing the weight gained in pregnancy. You will burn calories in the production and provision of breast milk. Breast milk, your baby's food source, comes from your calorie intake, is the perfect combination of nutrients premixed and packaged at the right temperature, requires no bottles, and is portable, going anywhere you go. And research indicates that breast-fed babies may be less apt to become obese in later life and less susceptible to allergies and chronic diseases such as heart disease than bottle-fed babies.

If your weight gain is the result of pregnancy, PMS is not an issue for you, and you're not near menopause, move on to Step Two on page 222.

Weight Gain and Menopause

Technically, menopause is defined as your last menstrual period, but the months and years leading up to it can be a "long good-bye." The menopausal transition is an interval of dynamic change that may begin as early as your late thirties or early forties but most often in your fifties. It may include uncomfortable symptoms, partially attributable to hormone fluctuations and possibly exacerbated by poor food choices and habits.

More women report weight gain as their major problem of menopause than any other symptom. The average weight gain from menopause to two years postmenopause reported in the *American Journal of Public Health* was 8 pounds. This did not include weight gained during the perimenopausal period that may have layered on additional pounds in advance of menopause.

In all women, the decline of estrogen changes the distribution of body fat. Whereas estrogen directs fat storage to the hips and thighs during the

Common Symptoms of Menopause: Irregular menses, irritability, hot flashes, night sweats, fatigue, trouble sleeping, feeling blue, inability to concentrate, forgetfulness, vaginal dryness, urine leakage, lower libido (sex drive), and weight gain.

first part of a woman's life, its declining profile sends excess weight to the midriff. This is termed *android obesity,* the *apple shape,* or what Paula calls the "menopot." Decreasing levels of estrogen may also cause the typical menopausal discomforts detailed on the previous page.

Shifts in metabolism, the rate at which calories burn, are also part of the pound-gathering picture. According to research reported in *The Journal of Clinical Endocrinology & Metabolism,* metabolism slows with age. As a result, women have to work harder after menopause to get the weight off and keep it off. The enzyme *adipose tissue lipoprotein lipase* (AT-LPL) is always at work in the body, preparing fat for uptake. It may also store fat in fat cells where you don't want it, more than ever after your estrogen drops in postmenopause. Furthermore, *lipolysis,* the action that releases fat from fat cells for use as fuel, diminishes by 75 percent during this life passage. With lethargic lipolysis and beefed-up AT-LPL activity, no wonder fat makes itself at home. The metamorphosis in body shape is one of the most disturbing changes occurring during menopause because it doesn't subside with time. Good thing diet and exercise can change that!

No matter what your age or phase of life, you don't have to live forever with hormone havoc and sporadic eating crazes. We no longer have to accept added pounds as a fact of being a female. Women can counterattack. Deploying specific eating strategies and making tactical food choices can prevent hormonal weight gain. Not only that; by making deliberate changes, you can begin to shed excess weight immediately. You'll feel notably better, both physically and mentally.

STEP TWO: KEEPING A FOOD RECORD

Don't think you can skip this step. Keeping a Food Record is one of the most important things you can do for yourself in following the Phenotype H Diet. Your first task is to log your cravings so you become aware of the way hormonal changes during PMS, pregnancy, or menopause affect your eating habits. Your Food Record should include what you crave, what you eat, how much you eat, and your hormonal state. Until you are aware of your patterns and can see them in black and white, it's very difficult, almost impossible, to change your habits. The Food Record will help you focus on what you're doing now that may be contributing to your weight. Here's an example of a Food Record page to get you started.

This isn't a time to delude yourself. If you swallow it, write it down. Writing down what you eat, meal after meal, day after day, will help you change your eating habits. If you aren't truthful with yourself, you won't see the patterns between your fluctuating hormones and the food you eat.

CRAVINGS AND FOOD RECORD

Date/Time	Location	Cravings	Food/Beverages Consumed	Amount	Hormonal State (i.e., PMS, pregnant, HRT use, or menopause transition)

This is not only eye-opening, it's life-changing work you're doing. When you face the truth of your behaviors, you not only become accountable, you become responsible for what, why, and when you eat. It may be shocking or embarrassing at first, so keep your Food Record in a safe, private place. Stick with it. The payoff will be a healthier, happier, and thinner you. After you have kept your Food Record for about a month, take some time to study it. Do you see a pattern? Are you having cravings right before your period, or are they tied to hormone use? Are you going through the menopausal transition and craving sweets or salt? Checking the patterns weekly will tell the story of your progress.

Sheila's story

"Biggie size equals biggie butt and biggie thighs."

"I'm on hormone patches because I had a hysterectomy when I was in my early thirties. Every time I change the patch, I crave carbs—especially chocolate, but most any sweets will do. It's taken time for me to figure this out and realize what I was doing. At first the hormone dose was too strong, and it really affected my outlook on life and my moods. Life would be great one minute and absolutely stink the next. I also felt very bloated, and you could definitely see the fluid buildup in my hands and under my eyes. I <u>always</u> looked tired and puffy.

"Over time and several changes in dose and form (pill to patch), I finally found one that works for me. But even now, I still do tend to crave chocolate and other sweet carbs at the time the new patch is applied, although the desire is much less than it used to be. As consistent a delivery system as the patch is, my desire (sometimes 'got to have it attitude') is definitely tied to my hormone levels.

"Regularly consuming these extra calories, plus sitting on my duff a lot of the time, and you have a recipe for back-end expansion and rolls under the bra strap. I had to take a step back and look hard at what I was doing and make changes.

"Food is everywhere we go. I can honestly tell you that getting weight off and keeping it off takes a serious commitment to cutting portions in our biggie-size world and getting way more exercise. One of my friends jokingly told me, 'Biggie size equals biggie butt and biggie thighs', and is she ever right!

"I have found what works for me (after a lot of trials) is the Phenotype H Diet plus a mix of yoga, Pilates, weight training, and swimming or other aerobic workout. When I had foot surgery a couple of years ago, my husband told me about the UBE [upper-body ergometer]. It gives you a great upper body cardio workout. Because I get bored easily, I vary my routine each week and make exercise fun—that way I want to do it. There's a great YMCA close to our home, and I take advantage of their terrific classes. Several of my girlfriends also go to the Y, and we try to meet for Pilates and yoga. We use e-mail to remind each other.

"The way I feel afterwards is so worth the juggling it takes to make it happen in my schedule. I set appointment times in my calendar for workouts, just like I do for any other client. It's true, it does take way more effort with each decade of life to stay fit, but once you make the decision to change, it becomes the way you live."

STEP THREE: DEVELOPING POSITIVE NONFOOD WEIGHT LOSS TRIGGERS

Just being a woman instead of a man may already be a genetic prescription for weight gain tied to hormones. As you now know from the "Understand Your Phenotype" section, you have probably inherited the propensity for weight problems from other women in your ancestry. Nonetheless, better habits can help you avoid the fat fate. The Phenotype H Diet detailed later in this chapter changes the three food-related negative triggers from the Weight Trigger Quiz into positive triggers: best food choices, structured meals, and controlled portions. The non-food-related ideas that follow complement and help you make the most of this dietary regime.

How did you score on the Weight Trigger Quiz's nonfood categories: "Stress," "No Regular Exercise," and "Increasingly Sedentary Lifestyle"? Melissa attributed her seven out of ten "true" answers in the "Stress" category to her incredibly stressful job as an emergency room nurse. Too much screen time made Sheila's sedentary lifestyle her main trigger. Neither they nor Samantha nor Paula got regular exercise.

With hormonal changes raising the likelihood of weight gain, you must fight back with deliberate changes to increase your metabolic rate and deal with stress. We recommend making one change like this at a time and letting it become a habit before you start the next change. It typically takes three to four weeks for a change to become part of your life. Set nonfood incentives, and reward yourself as you progress. Have a look at other strategies for turning off your greatest weight gain triggers.

Reduce Your Stress

Stress is the number one cause of diet relapses, and America's preponderance of fast and prepared foods—mostly high fat, high sodium, and highly processed—make it all too easy to blow your diet when the pressure is on, as it is during hormone-laced days or weeks. When you examine the episodes of sporadic eating and food craving in your Phenotype H Food

Record, you will notice, as Samantha did, that planning what to eat, rather than grabbing food on the move, could reduce both your weight and your stress level. The NO-TIME Menus gave Samantha examples of easy, quick meals, a way to manage her stress by changing her routines.

- Plan meals ahead, and have food ready to go. If you have time to cook on the weekends, make big pots of Tailgate Chili or other one-dish meals for use during the week. If you have to stop on the way home, try the grocery store rather than a fast-food place. Grab a rotisserie chicken and a bag of salad or other bagged veggies ready for the microwave.
- Create a list of enjoyable distractions, and during tense times busy yourself with them instead of munching. You can also use them as rewards. Melissa loves to visit yard sales and antique stores as a treat.
- Set aside a regular worry time. Samantha found that she worried all the time if she didn't plan a time to focus on her problems and talk them over with her husband. During the week, they began talking about the day as they shared a cup of decaf tea or flavored coffee. When stress tempts you to overeat or keeps you awake, remember to save those worries until your scheduled worry time.
- If you do lapse, please don't give up. Melissa reported that sometimes she does give in to her chocolate cravings; however, by limiting herself to the two fists of "Sweets, Treats, and Alcohol" weekly, she can manage both her cravings and her weight. By changing her attitude from "I blew the diet" to "This is a legal treat and not a problem," Melissa found she could control the amounts she ate even with PMS hormonal shifts.
- Make eating a conscious and deliberate event, not something you do when you're stressed. Paula found that if she kept low-fat yogurt, string cheese, or peanut butter crackers at work, she could always eat on time, fit them into her diet, and stave off the cravings that sometimes seemed to happen for no reason. For Samantha, scheduling meals allowed her not to be hungry and stopped the constant need to graze throughout the day.
- Replace any "unconscious eating" you may be doing while driving, watching TV, or working at the computer with a noncalorie liquid such as water or unsweetened tea. This way you will train yourself to make eating a different and distinct activity.

Develop an Active Lifestyle

At the end of a long day, Samantha used to turn on the TV while getting the kids something to eat. She would then sink into the couch along with the kids and eat whatever she could find in the kitchen or whatever they had picked up on the way home. Samantha needed strategies to prevent the sitting still and the hand-to-mouth habit that accompanied it. Waiting to turn on the TV until after dinner made eating an activity of its own. In addition, deliberate changes toward more activity, such as the following, are needed.

- Turn off the television or computer at least three nights a week and plan other activities.
- Take regular breaks when sitting at work for long periods of time, as Paula does, to stretch and drink water.
- Walk everywhere you can—even if it's outside with the dog a few times a day or out to get the mail or to a coworker's office rather than using the phone or e-mail. Get up and move.

Exercise Regularly

Don't believe diets that tell you that losing weight can be done without exercise. What they forget to mention is that keeping it off without exercise is virtually impossible. Women who exercise regularly find improvement in all hormone-related symptoms of PMS. It is not the intensity of exercise but the frequency that decreases the negative mood and physical symptoms. The beneficial effect of exercise is thought to come from decreasing the circulating brain chemicals associated with stress (epinephrine and norepinephrine), improving glucose tolerance, and elevating endorphin levels, those feel-good-about-yourself, happy hormones. So make time to exercise. This is especially helpful for women during the two weeks before their period.

In addition to its other benefits, exercise deflates stress, prevents boredom, and revs up metabolism for hours after the activity. For hormonal eaters, a daily workout will help put structure in your life and reduce sporadic eating.

- When you have the urge to eat, use exercise as one of your enjoyable distractions. Keep trying activities until you find an exercise you enjoy or will do routinely.
- Add frequent short bouts of exercise, such as 10 minutes at a time. Break the routine of sporadic eating with mini-exercises several times a day. Most people can walk away from their desk and go

somewhere—anywhere—to add activity during a long workday. Put on your pedometer and walk around your building or block, and watch the steps add up.

- Find a buddy to exercise with on a routine basis. Make appointments as Sheila did to meet a friend at the YMCA or fitness center or to take a walk in the neighborhood. Use e-mail to remind each other.

- Count your progress by using a pedometer regularly, as Melissa does. Although she is constantly on her feet in the ER, walking outside allows her mile-a-minute mind to unwind and think about other things, reducing her stress and giving her a needed break. You can buy a pedometer at sporting goods stores or order online from a site such as www.digiwalker.com or www.accusplit.com. Wear it daily so you can see how far you currently walk. Set a goal to increase your distance by at least 100 steps each day. You'll be surprised how motivating it is. Some pedometers even show how many calories you are burning! A positive trigger, counting steps increases your personal motivation, reinforcing new eating habits with more efficient metabolism and improved mood.

For many of you, these changes can easily be made on your own. But we know that for some of you these may seem like dramatic or even impossible changes. Because of their importance in changing your gene-based risks, please don't hesitate to seek help from a professional, such as a registered dietitian, licensed mental health professional, physician, or certified personal trainer.

STEP FOUR: FOLLOWING THE PHENOTYPE H DIET

Say good-bye to the weight gain and hormonal shifts that have too often felt as though they were pushing you to the edge. The Phenotype H Diet helps you get rid of your weight gain frustrations for good, whether they are the result of postpregnancy weight gain, PMS, or menopause. You will do this as you stop feeding your genetic predisposition to hormone-driven problems. You will replace your sporadic overeating and craving-led lapses with foods that nurture the woman in you. Thus, the diet will turn your food-based weight triggers into weight loss triggers with a specific food list, structured meals, and portion control. This plan will change the person you are on a cellular level and ensure you a much healthier future.

The Phenotype H Diet will:

- Help control your hormonal cravings so you can lose weight.
- Increase your intake of water and other fluids.
- Add diuretic foods to help relieve hormonal bloat.
- Add calcium-rich foods to aid in weight loss.
- Include seafood twice a week for mood stability.
- Include an afternoon snack for energy and mood control.
- Get rid of excess sodium to control fluid retention.

Focus Foods

The Phenotype H Diet has certain foods that are critical to your success. They're called Focus Foods because research has shown them to be specifically beneficial to hormonal eaters.

Water: Many women think that drinking lots of water will make them retain fluid, when actually it's just the opposite. Drinking adequate water helps maintain the body's balance of electrolytes (sodium, potassium, chloride) by flushing out the excess through urination. In other words, if you've eaten a lot of salty foods at a meal, drinking water works with the kidneys to get rid of the excess sodium. It's a good thing to do.

How much do you need? Your body contains about 10 to 12 gallons of water, which is equal to about 55 to 75 percent of your body weight. Generally, you need to drink a half ounce of water per pound of body weight. So a 130-pound person would require 65 ounces, or roughly 8+ cups per day—plus more when you exercise. Besides water, almost any nonalcoholic fluid counts toward your total.

Diuretic foods: Many foods have a very high water content that gives them a mild diuretic effect. Include fruits and vegetables that naturally contain a high percentage of water in your diet.

High-water-content fruits and vegetables: apple, asparagus, banana, blackberries, blueberries, broccoli, Brussels sprouts, cantaloupe, carambola (star fruit), cabbage, carrots, cauliflower, celery, cherries, cucumber, endive, grapefruit, grapes, green beans, lettuce, mushrooms, okra, onions, orange, parsley, peppers, pineapple, spinach, summer squash, tomato, watermelon

LIMIT YOUR SALT INTAKE

The recommended sodium intake is about 2,400 to 4,000 mg per day for women. However, it is not difficult to go over this amount, particularly when hormone fluctuations make you crave salty food. The problem is that salty food increases water retention and leads to bloating. Curbing your salt intake can diminish the water retention and bloating. A third of your sodium comes from what you add in cooking or at the table, so that's a good place to start limiting yourself. About two thirds of what you consume is added to processed food. The most common culprits are highly processed, ready-to-eat foods such as frozen dinners, chips, and other snack foods. By substituting low-sodium fresh fruits and vegetables and seasoning with herbs, garlic, and other seasonings instead of table salt you will quickly reduce water weight and that bloated feeling.

SODIUM FACTS: WHAT DOES THE LABEL MEAN?

LABEL DESCRIPTION	WHAT IT MEANS IN TERMS OF SODIUM LEVELS
Sodium free or salt free	Less than 5 mg per serving
Very low sodium	35 mg or less of sodium per serving
Low sodium	140 mg or less of sodium per serving
Reduced or less sodium	At least 25% less sodium than the regular version
Light in sodium	50% less sodium than the regular version
Unsalted or no salt added	No salt added to the product during processing

Calcium foods (milk, yogurt, cheese): Calcium-rich foods such as dairy products can help you lose weight, as numerous studies have confirmed. Recent studies reported in *The Journal of Nutrition* that people who consume less calcium, specifically from food, tend to be overweight and have greater midlife hormonally related weight gain. Fully 90 percent of women do not achieve the recommended calcium intake per day. Six hundred mg is the average for women, for whom calcium is extremely important to maintain bone density and strength. Studies associate each 300 mg daily intake of calcium (for example, 1 cup of low-fat yogurt) with up to 6 pounds weight loss per year. And when two people consumed the same number of calories in a day, the person who consumed 1,000 mg of calcium from dairy foods lost more weight and fat than the one who consumed only 600 mg.

As mentioned, calcium is an important electrolyte, helping to maintain a healthful balance of fluids in your system. In addition, high-calcium diets inhibit *lipogenesis,* fat-producing gene expression, and accelerate *lipolysis,* the breakdown of stored fat. By increasing the metabolic rate (the rate at which calories are burned), diets high in calcium further reverse fat storage and prevent weight gain.

Adding dairy foods to your diet is easy with all of the prepackaged yogurt smoothies, cheese sticks, and flavored milks in the grocery stores, or try a latte with skim milk for your midmorning coffee. In addition to dairy sources of calcium, soy products with calcium, orange juice and breakfast cereals fortified with calcium, and sardines and canned salmon with bones are good selections.

Seafood: The mood benefits of omega-3 fats come almost entirely from eicosapentaenoic acid (EPA) and docosahexaenoic acid (DHA), which are most concentrated in fatty fish such as salmon, tuna, and mackerel. If you have never eaten much fish or seafood, now is a good time to try. Tuna comes in easy-to-use pouches that can be mixed with some chopped apple and a little light mayonnaise to make a great minimeal. If you do not eat fish, fish oil supplements containing omega-3 fatty acids have been shown to have similar mood-stabilizing properties.

Alpha-linolenic acid–rich foods: The most abundant omega-3 fatty acid is alpha-linolenic acid (ALA), which is found in canola oil, soybeans, wheat germ, soybean oil, flaxseed, walnuts, and fish. The human body converts ALA into DHA and EPA, but in only modest amounts of about 5 to 15 percent. If you are a vegetarian or don't like seafood, you may still get some benefits by adding ALA sources daily, such as canola oil, soybeans, wheat germ, ground flaxseed, and walnuts. These are Focus Foods, too.

Flaxseed meal: Flaxseed is a great source of ALA. One table-spoon equals 1,500 milligrams ALA. In addition, flaxseed contains naturally occurring plant chemicals called phytochemicals and a good amount of fiber. That same tablespoon (about 60 calories), presently considered a safe and reasonable amount, will give you 3.3 grams of fiber, which is well on the way to the recommended 25+ grams per day. Dietary fiber delays stomach emptying and helps give you a feeling of fullness. It also acts a bit like a sponge in the body to help soak up and remove excess cholesterol. This is especially important for postmenopausal women, who are at greater risk for heart disease than are premenopausal women.

Here are some easy ways to add flaxseed meal to the diet:

- Stir into yogurt
- Sprinkle on hot cereal or fresh fruit
- Add to a smoothie recipe
- Stir into a bread, muffin, or pancake batter
- Mix in with granola
- Add to burgers, meat loaf, or casseroles

Soy: Soy contains isoflavones, which are a type of phytoestrogen or plant estrogen similar in their chemical makeup to human estrogen. Clinical trials are split on the benefit of isoflavones in combating night sweats, hot flashes or flushes, and vaginal dryness. Most research suggests that a trial of soy foods such as edamame (soybeans), soy nuts, tofu, and soy milk to see if they provide any relief for menopausal symptoms. One to two servings of soy food per day, containing a total of 60 to 100 mg of isoflavones, is the general recommendation unless you are directed otherwise by your doctor. Sometimes a combination of therapies, such as incorporating soy, getting more sleep, and finding ways to reduce stress, as well as improving your overall diet, can make a difference in your symptoms.

FOCUS FOOD FREQUENCY

FOOD ITEM	FREQUENCY
Water/fluids	Minimum of 64 ounces or 8 cups per day
Diuretic foods	Daily
Calcium-rich dairy foods	3–4 servings daily
Seafood	2–3 times per week
Walnuts	3 times per week
Wheat germ	1 tablespoon 3 times per week
Canola or soybean oil	Daily when oil is needed
Flaxseed, ground into meal	1 tablespoon 3 times per week
Soy foods	For menopause, try 1–2 servings per day

Begin with the Phenotype H *FAST TRACK* Two Weeks

With its quick results, the *FAST TRACK* Two Weeks gets you motivated to keep going. The *FAST TRACK* is too severe for achieving long-term changes to your phenotype, but it will jump-start your weight loss. You'll begin to feel leaner, healthier, and sexier within days. It uses the same format as the Phenotype H Diet below, with the following exceptions:

1. Omit the number of proteins, carbohydrates, and fats from the Phenotype H Diet, as **boldfaced** in parentheses in the Meals and Snack on the next page.
2. Omit the two fist-size 🖐 🖐 portions of "Sweets, Treats, and Alcohol" (see page 237) allowed each week.
3. Take a multivitamin/mineral supplement as well as the recommended additional vitamin C and vitamin E daily (see "Supplements" on page 240).
4. Start Week 3 with the full Phenotype H Diet.

THE PHENOTYPE H DIET

Select your foods for each meal and snack from the Food List on page 235. Sample Menus using foods that fit the diet are on page 238.

Meal 1
1 Protein (any fist, ½ fist, or thumb[s] selection)
2 Carbohydrates **(omit 1 carbohydrate for *FAST TRACK* Two Weeks)**
Freebie beverages

Meal 2
2 Proteins (1 palm **or** any 2: fist, ½ fist, or thumb[s] selections)
    (omit 1 protein for *FAST TRACK* Two Weeks)
2 Carbohydrates
Freebie vegetables
2 Fats **(omit 1 fat for *FAST TRACK* Two Weeks)**
Freebie beverages

Snack
1 Carbohydrate
1 Fat
Freebie beverages

Meal 3
2 Proteins (any 2: fist, ½ fist, or thumb[s] selections)
2 Carbohydrates
Freebie vegetables
3 Fats **(omit 1 fat for *FAST TRACK* Two Weeks)**
Freebie beverages

Stopped losing weight? Refer to "How to Deal with Plateaus" on page 28 and reboot your diet with another *FAST TRACK* Two Weeks.

FOOD LIST

Focus Foods are in **bold type.**

How much of each food should you eat? Use your hand as your guide. Eat the amount that you see; that is, the size of your fist, your palm, or your thumb.

 PALM

 FIST

 THUMB

Protein Sources

 Seafood. Poultry or lean meat. Poultry without skin, or lean cuts of meat such as loin, round, or cutlets of beef, pork, ham, veal, venison, lamb, etc., cook by steaming, sautéing, broiling, or grilling. Meat alternative (tofu, tempeh, or other soy product)

 Skim milk, buttermilk, evaporated skim milk, low-fat yogurt, low-fat cottage cheese, calcium-fortified soy milk, eggs such as Eggland's Best Eggs that are rich in omega-3 fatty acids (100 mg per egg), ricotta cheese (fat free)

½ **Edamame,** garbanzo, pinto, kidney, black, lima, or white beans; split, black-eyed, or field peas; lentils

  Parmigiano-Reggiano, grana padana, string cheese, Neufchâtel (reduced fat-cream cheese), soy cheese, walnuts, peanut butter, almond butter or other nut butters, almonds, Brazil nuts, cashews, chestnuts, hazelnuts, macadamia nuts, mixed nuts, peanuts, pecans, pine nuts, pistachios, **soy nuts,** pumpkin seeds, sunflower seeds

 Swiss, Cheddar, mozzarella, Romano, colby, feta, Gorgonzola, goat, or Monterey Jack cheese

Carbohydrate Sources

Whole grain bread, corn tortilla, whole wheat tortilla, whole grain English muffin or bagel, focaccia bread, whole wheat pita or ½ round whole grain lavash, whole grain crackers, corn bread, polenta, whole grain muffins, whole grain waffles or pancakes

Popped popcorn

High-fiber cereal, muesli

Apple, banana, berries, carambola (star fruit), cherries, citrus, grapes, kiwi fruit, **melon,** mango, nectarine, peach, pear, pineapple, plum

100% fruit juice, plain or calcium-fortified (limit to once a day)

½   Grits; oatmeal; Wheatena; couscous; whole wheat pasta, pasta with at least 2 grams of fiber per serving; brown rice or other whole grain; garbanzo, pinto, kidney, black, lima, or white beans; split, black-eyed, or field peas; lentils; **edamame;** corn; green peas; potatoes with skin; acorn or butternut squash; sweet potatoes or yams; plantain

Dried fruit such as raisins, cherries, blueberries, apricots, plums, figs, etc.

> Check out the *Freebie* list for lots of veggies, including salad greens, tomatoes, carrots, etc., that you don't have to limit.

Flaxseed meal, wheat germ

Fat Sources

MONOUNSATURATED FATS

Avocado, olives, hummus, almonds, Brazil nuts, cashews, chestnuts, hazelnuts, macadamia nuts, mixed nuts, peanuts, pecans, pine nuts, pistachios, **soy nuts, walnuts,** pumpkin seeds, safflower seeds, sesame seeds, sunflower seeds

Olive oil, canola oil, peanut oil, tahini paste, low-trans-fat margarines such as Olivio

POLYUNSATURATED FATS

🥄 🥄 Benecol Light or Take Control Light spread, light margarine, light mayonnaise, light salad dressing, low-trans-fat margarines such as Smart Balance

🥄 Benecol or Take Control spread, corn oil, safflower oil, soybean oil, sesame oil, sunflower oil, tartar sauce, salad dressing

Freebies

Beverages: Coffee, tea, diet soft drinks, **club soda, carbonated or mineral water**

For PMS: Decaf coffee, decaf tea, or diet soft drinks, **club soda, carbonated or mineral water**

Veggies: Artichoke, artichoke hearts, **arugula, asparagus,** bean sprouts, beets, **Bibb lettuce, broccoli, Brussels sprouts, carrots, cauliflower, cabbage, celery,** collard greens, **cucumber, endive, eggplant, escarole, green beans,** green onions or scallions, **green, red, or yellow pepper,** kale, kohlrabi, leeks, **lettuce, mixed greens, mesclun, mushrooms,** mustard greens, **okra, onions,** pea pods, radishes, **romaine, spinach, summer squash, tomato,** turnips, turnip greens, water chestnuts, **zucchini**

Miscellaneous: Broth or bouillon, ketchup, horseradish, lemon juice, lime juice, mustard, pickles, soy sauce, taco sauce, salsa, vinegars, garlic, fresh or dried herbs, pimento, spices, wine used in cooking, Worcestershire sauce, sugar substitutes

Sweets, Treats, and Alcohol

Okay, we know what you're thinking: "So where's my York Peppermint Patty and Chubby Hubby ice cream? Where is my wine?" The Phenotype H Diet allows you two fists 🍷 🍷 to use, as you desire. To use the two fists 🍷 🍷 as treats, you don't have to subtract anything from the Phenotype H Diet. You may use them both at once, such as on a slice of that heavenly dark chocolate torte with a raspberry glaze that you adore from the small café near your house, or split them up. That's the beauty of it—it's your choice. By allowing these treats (including alcohol), you're much less likely to feel deprived and want to run out and eat all those things you're trying to cut back on.

The food choices will be different for each person. They allow you the flexibility of having some "treats" and forestalling the deprivation-overeating cycle that can occur following a diet with no

To use the two fists 🍗 🍗 as treats, you don't have to subtract anything from the Phenotype H Diet.

treats. This helps you learn to get around the black-and-white thinking of "I'm on a diet or I'm off a diet." We have clients who get together with friends each week to indulge in their treats. This way they support one another and plan ahead to have something fun or slightly decadent. It keeps you in the real world of eating and enjoying food. These calories were already included in the calculations. Remember to include *everything* you eat in your journal.

SAMPLE MENUS

On days when you're rushed, use the NO-TIME Menus. MORE-TIME Menus are for days when you can cook leisurely. The menus are also meant as a guide for eating out.

NO-TIME Menu H

MEAL 1

🥙 1 Odwalla Bar: Peanut Crunch **or**

🥙 1 Clif Bar: Chocolate Chip Peanut Crunch

Freebie Decaf coffee, decaf tea, or sparkling water

MEAL 2

1 Lean Cuisine: Jumbo Rigatoni

Freebie Green leaf lettuce with:

Some mineral waters, including San Pellegrino, Vittel, Perrier, and Evian, contain around 100 to 200 milligrams of calcium per liter (about 34 ounces), making it even easier to add calcium to the diet.

    Freebie vegetables

🥄 🥄 Vidalia onion dressing (light, such as Ken's)

A bottle of San Pellegrino or other *Freebie* beverages

S<small>NEAK</small>

 Dried cranberry and  walnut mix

Sparkling water with a twist of lemon or other *Freebie* beverages

M<small>EAL</small> 3

 Rotisserie chicken (from grocery store)

 Confetti Couscous with:

> *Freebie* Shredded carrots
>
> *Freebie* Chopped onions

To save time, buy carrots already shredded. Microwave shredded carrots and chopped onions in with the couscous.

Freebie Arugula salad with:

> Grated grana padana cheese
>
>   Almonds
>
> Orange olive oil such as Olio Santo blood orange olive oil from Williams-Sonoma
>
> *Freebie* Balsamic vinegar

Sparkling water with a slice of lime or other *Freebie* beverages

MORE-TIME Menu H

M<small>EAL</small> 1

½ Multigrain hot cereal with flaxseed and soy (such as Hodgson Mill) with:

> Dried red cherries
>
> Skim milk or low-fat soy milk
>
> Drizzle of Vermont maple syrup

Coffee, tea, or other *Freebie* beverages

MEAL 2

 Tailgate Chili (see MORE-TIME Recipes in Appendix C)

 Corn bread

Freebie Mixed greens with:

> *Freebie* Tomato wedges
>
>   Italian dressing (light)

Freebie vegetables

Bottle of chilled Evian or other *Freebie* beverages

SNACK

 Bartlett pear, sliced, with   toasted pecans

Sparkling water with a twist of orange or other *Freebie* beverages

MEAL 3

 Herb-Rubbed Pork Tenderloin (see MORE-TIME Recipes in Appendix C)

 Wild Mushroom Risotto (see MORE-TIME Recipes in Appendix C)

Freebie Sautéed spinach with fresh garlic (with a spritz of olive oil)

Lemon-infused Perrier or other *Freebie* beverages

Supplements

PMS

Calcium: Calcium is a mineral that has benefit for reducing PMS symptoms. A meta-analysis (research review) of calcium for the management of PMS reported that 1,200–1,600 mg per day is effective. However, it may take three months before significant differences in symptoms appear.

Magnesium: Women with PMS have been shown to have lower blood levels of the mineral magnesium than women without the symptoms. In a study reported in *Obstetrics and Gynecology,* magnesium supplements were found to improve premenstrual mood changes significantly when taken from day 15 of the cycle to the onset of menses. Another small study reported positive results in preventing menstrual migraines.

Chasteberry: From the chaste tree (*Vitex agnus castus*), chasteberry has long been used for the treatment of menstrual disorders. A recent double-blind study reported in the *British Medical Journal* that dry chasteberry extract was effective in alleviating symptoms of irritability, anger, headache, and breast tenderness. The herb appears to help normalize hormone fluctuations when taken during the two-week luteal phase of the menstrual cycle.

The German health authorities (Commission E) have approved the use of chasteberry for irregularities of the menstrual cycle, PMS, and breast tenderness. *If you are pregnant or breast-feeding, do not take chasteberry, as the herb may interfere with the production of prolactin, a hormone released by the brain to stimulate breast-feeding.*

Ginkgo biloba: Ginkgo biloba has been used to treat the fluid retention symptoms associated with PMS, such as breast tenderness and bloating. For instance, a double-blind placebo-controlled study published in *Revue Française de Gynécologie et d'Obstétrique* evaluated 143 women with PMS symptoms for at least three consecutive cycles. Each woman was given 80 mg of ginkgo extract twice daily or a placebo beginning on day 16 of the menstrual cycle. The treatment was continued until the fifth day of the next cycle and resumed again on day 16 of that cycle. The results showed significant improvement in breast tenderness *and* emotional symptoms among the women taking the gingko.

Gingko is thought to improve circulation by decreasing blood thickness and reducing platelet activation (stickiness). *Ginkgo should not be used if you are taking warfarin, aspirin, heparin or any other drug with anticoagulant or antiplatelet effects.*

POSTPREGNANCY

Fish oil: If you're dealing with postpartum depression and don't like seafood or are allergic to it, a supplement of fish oil is a reasonable option.

MENOPAUSE

Black cohosh: An herb native to North America, black cohosh has become a staple in Europe for the treatment of menopausal symptoms. (Studies have also looked at it for PMS, with no benefit found.) In June 2001, the American College of Obstetricians and Gynecologists *Practice Bulletin* stated, "Black cohosh may be helpful in the short term (less than or equal to 6 months) as treatment for vasomotor symptoms such as hot flashes or night sweats."

German health authorities (Commission E) have also endorsed the use of black cohosh for menopausal symptoms but do not recommend its use for longer than six months due to the lack of long-term safety data. The most common side effect is gastrointestinal discomfort. Remifemin is the brand that has been most extensively studied. *Black cohosh is not recommended for women with a family history of breast cancer or breast cancer survivors.*

Isoflavones: Common phytoestrogens found in soybeans are structurally similar to estradiol, which is a form of estrogen. In postmenopausal women, when estradiol is low or nonexistent, isoflavones may reduce symptoms such as hot flashes and night sweats. If you've tried all the new soy food products and cannot consume enough to make a difference, a short-term trial of an isoflavone supplement such as Nature Made Soy 50 or Healthy Woman is worth a try for relieving menopause symptoms. *Do not use without discussion with your physician if you have had estrogen-dependent breast cancer or have a strong family history of breast cancer.*

Valerian (*Valeriana officinalis*)**:** An herb that has been used for centuries for insomnia, valerian was approved as a sleep aid in Germany as early as 1985 and appears to be most useful when taken over time for chronic sleep problems. Its mechanism of action is not well understood, but it may affect the brain's production of gamma-amino butyric acid GABA, a chemical associated with reducing anxiety.

Studies have shown that it may take two to four weeks of regular use to produce significantly improved sleep. So if your sleeping problem is situational and lasts for a short time, for example, after a stressful incident that disrupts sleep for a night or two, valerian may not be much help. But if you have difficulty sleeping for months as you move from perimenopause to menopause, valerian may be worth a try. *It should not be used in addition to other medications for insomnia or antianxiety medications, such as benzodiazapenes (Ativan or Xanax).*

SUPPLEMENT
RECOMMENDATIONS AND DOSES

SUPPLEMENT	DOSE
ALL PHENOTYPE H WOMEN:	
Multivitamin/mineral	Daily
Vitamin C	250 mg daily
Vitamin E	200 IU mixed tocopherols daily
PMS:	
Magnesium	500–1,000 mg for PMS beginning on day 15 of the cycle and ending when the menstrual period begins
Calcium (citrate or carbonate)	1,200–1,600 mg daily in divided doses of not more than 500 mg each
Chasteberry	225–400 mg daily during the luteal phase of the menstrual cycle (2 weeks prior to menses)
Ginkgo biloba	160–240 mg daily in two or three divided doses

Severe PMS may require treatment with antidepressant medications. Selective serotonin reuptake inhibitors (SSRIs), such as Prozac, Paxil, and Sarafem, seem to provide the greatest benefit because they increase the production of serotonin. By raising their serotonin level, women reported reduced symptoms and improved functioning with only occasional side effects such as dry mouth or gastrointestinal upset.

These results were much better than treatment with a different class of antidepressant, the tricyclic group, which includes Tofranil and Elavil. The tricylic antidepressants don't limit their effects to serotonin but influence other neurotransmitters as well and thus are more prone to causing side effects than are the SSRIs.

(continued on next page)

SUPPLEMENT	DOSE
POSTPREGNANCY:	
Fish oil	1,000 mg capsule supplying 180 mg of EPA and 120 of DHA; take 3 times daily
MENOPAUSE:	
Black cohosh	1 tablet (typically 20 mg) twice daily
Isoflavones	60–100 mg daily
Valerian	1,000 mg of dried valerian root in tablet form taken 30–60 minutes before bedtime

The Phenotype H Maintenance Diet

Remember when you started on the Phenotype H Diet? In a few days, something inside just seemed to click and you began to lose weight, feel better, and feel healthier. That will not change.

Remember how overwhelmed Samantha was with her two children, her job, her hectic life, and her sporadic eating? That she examined her priorities and decided she had to take charge? Samantha learned that she enjoyed keeping other people's children. Day care has become her own small business, and she has made up for her old salary. She says, "I've become more assertive and like trying things I've never tried before." Samantha has also lost 40 pounds on the Phenotype H Diet and has kept it off by creating balance in her life.

When you reach your weight goal as Samantha did, you are ready to move on to the Phenotype H Maintenance Diet. The diet has the same backbone Focus Foods. Still tailored to your genetic blueprint, it will keep you satisfied and your weight constant. A high level of physical activity or exercise is the single best predictor of keeping lost weight off. So keep moving!

THE PHENOTYPE H MAINTENANCE DIET

Meal 1
1 Protein (any fist, ½ fist, or thumb[s] selection)
2 Carbohydrates
Freebie beverages

Meal 2
2 Proteins (1 palm **or** any 2: fist, ½ fist, or thumb[s] selections)
2 Carbohydrates
Freebie vegetables
2 Fats
Freebie beverages

Snack
1 Carbohydrate
1 Fat
Freebie beverages

Meal 3
2 Proteins (any 2: fist, ½ fist, or thumb[s] selections)
3 Carbohydrates
Freebie vegetables
4 Fats
Freebie beverages

No-Prep Foods

Here is a list of No-Prep foods to pick up at the grocery or convenience store. These are great when you don't have the time or place to fix something or can't sit down in a restaurant to eat. No-Prep means just that—open and eat. Be sure to think about the number of protein, carbohydrate, and fat servings on your diet plan for the meal or snack you choose.

You will have to estimate the correct portion size using your hand, as you have for all your foods on your phenotype food list. Product sizes vary all over the country. Your serving size is the amount allowed in terms of your hand size. Item location will vary by type of store.

 PALM

 FIST

 THUMB

Bakery

 Bagels (top with low-fat cream cheese or peanut butter)

 Raisin bran muffins (even better if made with liquid oil rather than hydrogenated oil)

Dairy/Alternatives

Blueberry smoothie (such as Odwalla)

Cheese sticks

DanActive probiotic dairy drink

Laughing Cow cheese (doesn't require refrigeration)

Milk chugs (single serving low-fat or skim milk)

Slim·Fast (check for cold ones in deli or drink case)

Snack size cottage cheese (such as Light n' Lively)

Soy drinks in smaller sizes such as

> Coffee soylatte

> Vanilla, chocolate

Yogurt cups, low-fat and one third fewer calories (less sugar)

Yogurt drinks (smoothies; there are so many of these that you must compare the labels to make the best choice,)

Yogurt tubes

Deli

Because these products vary greatly by store and recipe, one type of potato salad may have twice the fat of another choice. Compare your options and follow the portion guides, using your fist, palm, or thumb.

Freebie Bottled water or flavored water without calories

Carrot raisin salad

Deli baked beans

Fresh fruit cups

Garden pasta

Freebie Green tea or other tea (canned with nothing added)

Greek style salad

Hard-cooked eggs

Hummus and pita (such as Athenos Travelers)

Freebie Kosher garlic pickles

Macaroni salad

Pimento cheese

Potato salad

Red pepper hummus

Salata Mediterranean salad

Shredded coleslaw

Smoked salmon

Soup of the day (non–cream based) with corn bread or other whole grain bread

Subs and other sandwiches made with lean meats and topped with vegetables

Summer rolls (typically found with sushi)

Sushi

Taboule

Tropicana peach smoothie

Turkey salad

V8 juice with a lemon twist (there are several V8 flavors)

White tuna salad

Miscellaneous

Clif Bars, such as Crunchy Peanut Butter or Chocolate Chip Peanut Crunch

Granola or trail mix (ingredients really vary by brand, so compare them)

Gourmet baked chips such as Kettle Krisps or Guiltless Gourmet

Just Tomatoes and similar snacks, such as Just Mango, Just Raspberries, or Just Roasted Garlic

New York flat breads (crackers)

Nuts

Odwalla Bars such as Chocolate or Peanut Crunch

Peanut butter crackers

Peanut butter (also available in squeeze containers and individually wrapped slices)

Peanut butter–filled pretzels

Popcorn, light

Pop-top cans of fruit or individual fruit bowls

Pop-top tuna or tuna pouches

Powerbar: Harvest

Raisins and other dried fruit

Raspberry bars, such as Natural Choice

Soy crisps, such as Genisoy Zesty Barbecue (other salty and sweet varieties available)

Soynuts

🍪 Triscuits (reduced fat)

🍪 Whole Food's VERVE Bar, such as Peanut Butter Crunch or Chocolate Chip Peanut Crunch

Energy Bars

Energy bars, trail mix, and trail mix bars can be quite high in calories, so compare them. They can even vary within the same brand. For example, some may have a coating that contains hydrogenated fat, so pay close attention to the ingredients as well as the Nutrition Facts label.

THE BEST ENERGY BARS HAVE:

- At least 3 grams of fiber, preferably 5 or more
- Low saturated fat grams and sugar grams (1 teaspoon sugar = 4 grams)
- 7–10 grams of protein for women and up to 15 grams of protein for men if used to replace a minimeal or snack.
- No palm kernel oil, coconut oil, or trans fat, indicated by hydrogenated or fractionated fat

Produce

Freebie Baby carrots

Freebie Carrots and ranch dip (such as Coolcuts)

Freebie Celery with dip (found in produce section)

🖐 Cut-up fruit:

　　　Pineapple

　　　Honeydew

　　　Cantaloupe

　　　Watermelon

　　　Strawberries

🖐 Fruit by the piece

Freebie Garden salad in a to-go container

🖐 Grapes by the bunch

Freebie Spinach salad in a to-go container

🖐 Tropicana juice bottles (found with juice, usually by produce)

Ready Remedies

PANTRY REMEDIES

Brown rice, instant
Canned beans
Canned tomatoes, tomato paste, and tomato sauce
Canned tuna and/or salmon, water-packed
Canola and olive oil
Cereals: low sugar, high fiber
Crackers, whole grain
Garlic, fresh
Granola
Herbs, dried
Honey or maple syrup
Muffin mixes, no or very low in trans fat or hydrogenated fat
Nuts: slivered almonds, walnut halves, pecan halves, pine nuts,
    pistachios
Oats
Onions: purple and Vidalia
Pasta sauce
Pastas, whole wheat or with at least 2 grams of fiber per serving
Peanut butter
Popcorn, low fat (no trans fat) microwave
Potatoes, sweet and baking

Raisins, dried cherries, and dried apricots
Refried beans/vegetarian refried beans, fat free
Salsa
Soy sauce, low sodium
Tomatoes, sun-dried
Vegetable/chicken/beef broth: fat free, lower sodium
Vegetable oil cooking spray
Vinegars: balsamic, apple cider, and red wine
Wheat germ

REFRIGERATOR REMEDIES

Baby carrots
Eggs
Lemon and lime juices
Margarine or spread, no or very low trans fat
Mayonnaise, light
Milk, skim
Mustard
Olives: green, kalamata, and niçoise
Pizza dough or ready to use crust with no trans fat
Salad dressings, light
Salad mixes, bagged
Shredded cheese, low-fat
Sour cream, light
Tofu: firm and soft
Tortillas: corn and whole wheat or sprouted wheat
Yogurt: low-fat or nonfat
Vegetables, precut

FREEZER REMEDIES

Bagels, whole grain
Chicken breasts, boneless, skinless
Ground turkey breast/ground chicken breast/extra lean ground
    beef
Soy burgers
Soy crumbles
Strawberries, blueberries, and blackberries
Vegetables for stir-fry, pizza toppings, etc.
Waffles: whole grain, low-fat

FINDING FIRST-RATE FROZEN DINNERS

Look at the Nutrition Facts label and the ingredients:

- Total fat should be 30 percent or less of the daily value (DV) unless the majority of the fat is monounsaturated; then the total fat can go up to 40 percent.
- When comparing dinners, less is better for grams of saturated fat.
- When comparing dinners, look at the grams of fiber and the percentage of calcium. More is better.
- Check out dinners that include vegetables and/or whole grains such as Amy's Organics and Seeds of Change.
- To use as a minimeal, look for a dinner providing 300 calories or less for women, or 350 or less for men.
- To use as a meal replacement, look for a dinner providing 450 calories or less for women, or 500 or less for men.

Recipes

Who wants to eat "diet food" that is tasteless and unappealing, no matter how healthy it may be? To us, great taste and health go hand in hand. Food should feed and strengthen the body, certainly, but it should also look appealing and nourish the soul. We enjoy good food and we love to cook. We've used these recipes over and over. Some of these recipes are very simple and will quickly become weekly standards. Others take more time but the special result is worth the little extra effort in the kitchen. You can fix these dishes repeatedly for your family and friends, knowing they will love the meal and ask for the recipes. The recipes are grouped by phenotype based on the focus foods and other characteristics of each phenotype diet. That doesn't mean that they shouldn't be used for other phenotypes as well. Enjoy!

These recipes use the same serving sizes based on the hand as the phenotype food lists. Following each will be the serving size expressed as a palm, fist, or thumb(s).

 PALM

 FIST

 THUMB

PHENOTYPE A

NO-TIME Recipes

BALSAMIC-DILL VINAIGRETTE

PREP TIME: 5 MINUTES

¼ cup olive oil
3 tablespoons balsamic vinegar
1 tablespoon white distilled vinegar
1 tablespoon snipped fresh dill
2 teaspoons sugar (can use sugar substitute)
¼ teaspoon coarsely ground black pepper

Combine all ingredients in a small bowl; whisk vigorously.

Drizzle over fresh spring mix salad greens or toss into a pasta salad.

Yield: 8 servings
Serving size: 🥄 *= 1 fat*

PHYTO-FRUIT SMOOTHIE: NUT CASE

PREP TIME: 5 MINUTES

1 banana
1 cup low-fat vanilla frozen yogurt
2 tablespoons chocolate syrup
2 tablespoons peanut butter
5–6 ice cubes

Place all ingredients into a blender or food processor. Blend thoroughly.

Yield: approximately 2 servings
Serving size: 🥤 *= 1 protein, 3 carbohydrates, 1 fat*

VEGETABLE PASTA WITH ROASTED RED PEPPERS

PREP TIME: 5 MINUTES
COOK TIME: 8–10 MINUTES

6 ounces uncooked whole wheat fettuccine
1 medium zucchini, shredded
1 yellow squash, shredded
1 medium carrot, shredded
1 (4-ounce) package crumbled Gorgonzola cheese

1 roasted red pepper, thinly sliced
¼ teaspoon coarsely ground black pepper

Cook pasta according to package directions. Place zucchini, squash, and carrot in a colander; drain pasta over vegetables. Transfer both to a large bowl and add cheese, roasted pepper, and black pepper; toss gently.

Yield: 4 servings

Serving size: 👊 *= 1 protein (fist, ½ fist or thumb), 2 carbohydrates, Freebie vegetables*

MORE-TIME Recipes

SPICY CHICKEN BOLOGNESE OVER WHOLE WHEAT PASTA

PREP TIME: 20 MINUTES
COOK TIME: 60 MINUTES

Bolognese is a thick, meaty ragu or sauce typical of northern Italy. Whole wheat pasta is used in all of our pasta dishes for its nutty flavor, nutrition, and fiber content.

2 tablespoons olive oil
1 pound ground chicken breast
1 medium yellow onion, chopped
1 (8-ounce) bag shredded carrots
1 garlic clove, minced
½ cup dry white wine
1 (28-ounce) can crushed tomatoes in extra puree (can use lower sodium version)
1½ cups chicken broth (can use lower sodium version)
1 tablespoon chopped fresh parsley
¼ cup half-and-half
3 tablespoons chopped fresh basil
½ teaspoon salt (optional)
¼ teaspoon coarsely ground black pepper
6 cups hot cooked whole wheat angel hair or other pasta (about 12 ounces uncooked)
¼ cup freshly grated Parmigiano-Reggiano

Heat oil in a Dutch oven over medium heat. Brown the ground chicken with onion and carrots in the oil over medium-high heat. Add garlic; sauté 1 minute and add wine. Stir frequently until liquid is reduced by half. Stir

(continued on next page)

in tomatoes, broth, and parsley. Bring to a boil, reduce heat, and simmer uncovered 45 minutes, or until slightly thickened. Stir in half-and-half, basil, salt, and pepper; cook 5 minutes. Serve over pasta and top with cheese.

Yield: 6 servings

Serving size: 🍴 *= 1 protein, 3 carbohydrates, 1 fat,* Freebie *vegetables*

HORSERADISH ROASTED POTATOES

PREP TIME: 5 MINUTES
COOK TIME: 45 MINUTES

1 tablespoon olive oil
3 tablespoons prepared horseradish
1½ pounds small red potatoes, quartered (about 8 potatoes)

1. Preheat oven to 425°. Lightly coat a 13 x 9-inch baking dish with cooking spray.

2. In a large bowl combine olive oil and horseradish; add potatoes, tossing to coat. Transfer to baking dish; roast 45 minutes, or until tender, stirring occasionally.

Yield: 4 servings

Serving size: 🍴 *= 2 carbohydrates, 1 fat*

PORTOBELLO CHICKEN ENCHILADAS

PREP TIME: 15 MINUTES
COOK TIME: 35 MINUTES

1 cup chopped cooked skinless chicken breast (about 12 ounces)
1 (8-ounce) block Cabot 50% Light Jalapeno Cheddar, shredded
½ cup reduced-fat sour cream
1 (4½-ounce) can chopped green chilies, drained
½ cup chopped fresh cilantro
1 cup chopped portobello mushrooms
½ cup chopped red onion
4 (8-inch) flour tortillas (try whole wheat or sprouted wheat)

1. Preheat oven to 350°. Coat 8 x 8-inch baking dish with cooking spray.

2. Mix together the first seven ingredients (chicken through onion) in a large mixing bowl. Spoon mixture evenly down center of each tortilla; roll

up. Arrange seam side down in prepared baking dish. Coat tortillas with cooking spray; bake 35 minutes, or until golden brown.

3. Serve with diced tomatoes, jalapeños, ripe olives, avocado wedge, sliced green onions, cilantro, and/or salsa.

Yield: 4 servings

Serving size: ✍ *= 1 protein, 2 carbohydrates, 2 fats, Freebie vegetables*

PHENOTYPE B

NO-TIME Recipes

CHEDDAR AND ZUCCHINI BRUSCHETTE

PREP TIME: 15 MINUTES
COOK TIME: 5 MINUTES

1 teaspoon olive oil
1 medium zucchini, chopped
1 garlic clove, minced
¼ teaspoon salt
1 medium tomato, chopped
¼ teaspoon coarsely ground black pepper
1 cup (4 ounces) shredded Cabot 50% Light Cheddar
8 (½-inch-thick) slices crusty Italian bread, toasted

Heat oil in a large nonstick skillet over medium-high heat. Add zucchini, garlic, and salt; sauté 2 minutes. Add tomato and pepper; sauté 2 minutes. Transfer mixture to medium bowl; stir cheese into zucchini mixture. Mound 1 heaping tablespoon on each slice of toast. Serve warm.

Yield: 8 servings

Serving size: ✍ *= 1 protein (fist, ½ fist, or thumb), 1 carbohydrate,*
Freebie vegetables

CHERRY-BANANA TOSS WITH ORANGE ITALIAN DRESSING

PREP TIME: 5 MINUTES

8 cups spring salad mix
½ cup walnut pieces
½ cup dried cherries or dried cranberries
½ cup crumbled Gorgonzola
1 banana, sliced

(continued on next page)

Place salad mix in a large bowl. Add walnuts, cherries, and cheese to salad mix; toss gently. Divide evenly among four salad plates. Slice banana and add to salad just before serving. Drizzle with Orange Italian Dressing.

Yield: 8 servings

Serving size: 👌 🍴 *= 1 protein (fist, ½ fist, or thumb), 2 carbohydrates, Freebie vegetables, plus 1 fat for dressing (see below)*

Orange Italian Dressing

PREP TIME: 5 MINUTES

¼ cup fresh orange juice with pulp
2 tablespoons extra virgin olive oil
1 tablespoon sugar (can use sugar substitute)
1 heaping tablespoon orange marmalade
1 tablespoon balsamic vinegar
1 tablespoon snipped fresh dill
¼ teaspoon coarsely ground black pepper

Combine all ingredients; whisk vigorously.

Yield: 8 servings

Serving size: 👍 *= 1 fat*

CLASSIC SALMON WITH CONFETTI VEGETABLES

PREP TIME: 10 MINUTES
COOK TIME: 10 MINUTES

Our friend Becky frequently makes this recipe for guests. The edamame, a good protein source, is a terrific twist.
Tip: You can find edamame in the freezer section with the vegetables.

½ cup orange juice
½ cup diced yellow squash
½ cup diced zucchini
½ cup diced unpeeled sweet potato
½ cup diced unpeeled eggplant
½ cup frozen shelled edamame (green soybeans)
2 (4- to 6-ounce) salmon fillets (about 1 inch thick)
2 teaspoons grated peeled fresh ginger

Combine the first six ingredients (orange juice through edamame). Heat large skillet over medium-high heat; add vegetable mixture and salmon.

Cover and steam 10 minutes, or until fish flakes easily when tested with a fork. Serve topped with grated ginger.

Yield: 2 servings

Serving size: ✺ salmon = 1 protein, 1 fat;

✊ vegetables = 1 carbohydrate; Freebie vegetables

GRAPEFRUIT AND KIWI SALAD WITH POPPY SEED DRESSING
PREP TIME: 10 MINUTES

Tip: To make orange peel curls, cut 6-inch strips of orange peel with a vegetable peeler and curl them around the end of a wooden spoon until the peel holds its shape.

    4 Boston lettuce leaves
    2 grapefruits, peeled and sectioned
    2 kiwis, peeled and sliced
    ½ cup raspberries
    4 orange peel curls (optional)

Arrange lettuce and fruits evenly among four plates. Drizzle each with Poppy Seed Dressing and garnish with orange curls, if desired.

Yield: 4 servings

Serving size: ✊ = 1 carbohydrate plus 1 fat for dressing (see below).

Poppy Seed Dressing
PREP TIME: 3 MINUTES

Tip: The zest is the colorful skin of citrus fruit. Remove with a zester or grater.

    1 teaspoon grated orange zest
    ¼ cup fresh orange juice with pulp
    ¼ cup honey
    ¼ teaspoon poppy seeds

Combine all ingredients; whisk vigorously. Drizzle over salads.

Yield: 8 servings

Serving size: ✿ = 1 fat

ITALIAN PASTA WITH PLUM TOMATOES AND FRESH BASIL

PREP TIME: 7 MINUTES
COOK TIME: 12–14 MINUTES

1 tablespoon olive oil
3 plum tomatoes, sliced
6 large basil leaves, chopped
1 teaspoon minced garlic
¼ teaspoon salt
⅛ teaspoon coarsely ground black pepper
3 cups hot cooked whole wheat penne (about 6 ounces uncooked)

Heat oil in a medium nonstick skillet over medium-high heat. Lightly sauté tomatoes, basil, garlic, salt, and pepper. Add to pasta; toss gently.

Yield: 2 servings
Serving size: 1½ 🖐 = 2 proteins (fist, ½ fist, or thumb),
3 carbohydrates, 1 fat, Freebie vegetables

PHYTO-FRUIT SMOOTHIE: BERRY-BANANA COOLER

PREP TIME: 5 MINUTES

1 banana
1 cup frozen strawberries
1 cup low-fat vanilla frozen yogurt

Place all ingredients into a blender or food processor. Blend thoroughly.

Yield: approximately 2 servings
Serving size: 🖐 = 1 protein, 3 carbohydrates

PHYTO-FRUIT SMOOTHIE: LEMON SQUEEZER

PREP TIME: 5 MINUTES

1 banana
1 cup frozen raspberries
½ cup low-fat vanilla frozen yogurt
½ cup lemon sherbet

Place all ingredients into a blender or food processor. Blend thoroughly.

Yield: approximately 2 servings
Serving size: 🖐 = 4 carbohydrates

ZESTY GREEN BEANS

PREP TIME: 5 MINUTES
COOK TIME: 10 MINUTES

With a busy career and fairly long commute, Susan's friend Joye is always looking for fast yet tasty ways to prepare her fresh vegetables. You can substitute other vegetables for the green beans.

1½ pounds fresh green beans
1 small onion, chopped
¼ teaspoon salt or herb seasoning blend
¼ teaspoon coarsely ground black pepper
2 firm plum tomatoes, sliced
2 tablespoons chopped fresh basil
4 tablespoons light Italian dressing

Wash and snap beans to desired size, discarding stem ends. Combine beans, ⅓ cup water, onion, salt, and pepper in a microwavable dish. Cover and microwave on high 10 minutes, or until crisp-tender. Drain. Add tomatoes, basil, and dressing and toss gently.

Yield: 4 servings

Serving size: 🖐 *= 1 fat,* Freebie *vegetables*

MORE-TIME Recipes

CARROT CHOWDER WITH TURKEY

PREP TIME: 20 MINUTES
COOK TIME: 1–1¼ HOURS

This is hearty and a meal in itself! Look for lower-sodium versions of the tomato soup, broth, and stewed tomatoes if desired.

1 pound ground chicken or turkey
1½ teaspoons canola oil
2 medium onions, chopped
2 celery stalks, sliced
½ green pepper, chopped
2 (10¾-ounce) cans low-fat condensed cream of mushroom soup
1 (10¾-ounce) can condensed tomato soup
1 (16-ounce) can stewed tomatoes

(continued on next page)

> 3 cups chicken broth
> 3 yellow squash, sliced
> 2 (8-ounce) bags shredded carrots
> 8 ounces sliced fresh mushrooms
> ½ teaspoon coarsely ground black pepper

1. Brown chicken in a large Dutch oven over medium-high heat; remove and keep warm.

2. Heat oil in the same Dutch oven. Sauté onions, celery, and green pepper; drain. Return chicken to Dutch oven with onion mixture and add remaining ingredients (mushroom soup through pepper) and 1½ cups water. Bring to a boil; reduce heat and simmer until vegetables are tender, about 1–1¼ hours. Ladle soup into bowls.

Yield: 10 cups
Serving size: 🖐 *= 1 protein (fist, ½ fist, or thumb),*
1 carbohydrate, 1 fat, Freebie *vegetables*

CINNAMON-APPLESAUCE MUFFINS

PREP TIME: 20 MINUTES
COOK TIME: 10–12 MINUTES

Susan's Aunt Rachel shared this recipe. It makes 48 minimuffins with a big taste that freeze well and are great for snacks or breakfast.

> 2 cups all-purpose flour
> ½ teaspoon ground cinnamon
> ½ teaspoon salt
> 1 cup sugar
> ⅔ cup canola oil
> 1 teaspoon vanilla extract
> 1 teaspoon baking soda
> 1 cup applesauce, warmed
> ¾ cup raisins
> ½ cup chopped pecans

1. Preheat oven to 400°. Spray minimuffin pans with cooking spray or line with paper baking cups.

2. Stir together flour, cinnamon, and salt in a large bowl; set aside. Whisk together sugar, oil, and vanilla in medium bowl. Add baking soda to applesauce and combine with sugar mixture. Add wet mixture to dry mixture and stir just until moist. Stir in raisins and pecans.

3. Spoon 1 tablespoon batter into each muffin cup. Bake 10 to 12 minutes, or until wooden pick inserted in center comes out clean. Remove muffins from pan immediately; cool on wire racks.

Yield: 48 minimuffins

Serving size: 2 minimuffins; ½ 🏈 *= 1 carbohydrate, 1 fat*

GARLIC-CRUSTED CHICKEN WITH PECORINO ROMANO CHEESE
PREP TIME: 7 MINUTES
COOK TIME: 16 MINUTES

Susan's friend Carol has a large Italian family, and this recipe is a staple at their house. Carol always cooks extra chicken and slices the leftovers for sandwiches and to top salads.

Tip: She uses Benecol Light or Take Control Light spread in place of margarine.

2 cups dry Italian-seasoned bread crumbs
2 tablespoons grated Pecorino Romano or other Romano
2 tablespoons coarsely ground garlic powder with parsley
1 teaspoon coarsely ground back pepper
¾ cup egg substitute or 3 eggs
12 (4- to 6-ounce) skinless, boneless chicken breast halves
2 tablespoons margarine (low trans fat)

1. Preheat broiler. Coat a foil-lined baking sheet with cooking spray.

2. Combine bread crumbs, cheese, garlic powder, and pepper in a large bowl. Pour eggs into a separate large bowl. Dip chicken into eggs; dredge in bread crumb mixture and place on baking sheet. Spread chicken with half of the margarine; broil 6 inches from heat for 9 minutes. Turn chicken and spread with remaining margarine; broil 7 additional minutes, or until done.

Yield: 12 servings

Serving size: 🍗 *= 1 protein, 1 carbohydrate, 1 fat*

PHENOTYPE C

NO-TIME Recipes

MAPLE-GINGER SALMON

PREP TIME: 5 MINUTES
COOK TIME: 20 MINUTES

2 (4- to 6-ounce) salmon fillets (about 1 inch thick)
¼ teaspoon salt (optional)
¼ teaspoon coarsely ground black pepper
3 tablespoons maple syrup
2 tablespoons chopped peeled fresh ginger

Preheat oven to 450°. Coat a foil-lined pan with cooking spray. Place salmon skin side down on pan; sprinkle with salt and pepper. Combine syrup and ginger; brush salmon with half of the syrup mixture and bake 10 minutes. Brush on remaining half of syrup; bake an additional 7 minutes, or until fish flakes easily when tested with a fork.

Yield: 2 servings
Serving size: ▧ = 1 protein, 1 fat

PHYTO-FRUIT SMOOTHIE: MANGO MANIA

PREP TIME: 5 MINUTES

1 banana
1 cup fresh mango
1 cup pineapple sherbet
5–6 ice cubes

Place all ingredients into a blender or food processor. Blend thoroughly.

Yield: approximately 2 servings
Serving size: ▧ = 3 carbohydrates

PHYTO-FRUIT SMOOTHIE: PEACH MELBA

PREP TIME: 5 MINUTES

1 banana
1 cup raspberry sherbet
½ cup frozen sliced peaches
½ cup frozen raspberries

Place all ingredients into a blender or food processor. Blend thoroughly.

Yield: approximately 2 servings

Serving size: 🍴 *= 4 carbohydrates*

MORE-TIME Recipes

CATHY'S VEGETABLE SPAGHETTI SAUCE WITH FRESH GARLIC

PREP TIME: 15 MINUTES
COOK TIME: 1–1½ HOURS

Cathy makes this sauce when her husband's large family comes to visit. It serves 16, so make it when you expect a crowd. The leftover sauce freezes well in meal-size portions. It's a MORE-TIME Recipe that makes great NO-TIME Meals and the flavor just gets better. Look for lower-sodium versions of the tomato sauce, stewed tomatoes, and spaghetti sauce if desired.

1 tablespoon olive oil
5 garlic cloves, minced
1 large onion, chopped
1 green pepper, chopped
1 pound fresh mushrooms, sliced
3 (14½-ounce) cans tomato sauce
3 (14½-ounce) cans stewed tomatoes
1 (25-ounce) jar spaghetti sauce
2 (8-ounce) bags shredded carrots
2 teaspoons dried Italian seasoning
2 teaspoons dried oregano
2 bay leaves
¼ teaspoon coarsely ground black pepper
6 cups hot cooked whole wheat fettuccine (about 12 ounces uncooked)

Heat oil in a large saucepan over medium heat. Sauté garlic, onion, green pepper, and mushrooms for 1 minute. Add all remaining ingredients except fettucine. Bring to a boil; reduce heat, and simmer for 1–1½ hours. Discard bay leaves and serve over pasta.

Yield: 16 servings

Serving size: 🍴 *= 1 protein (fist, ½ fist, or thumb),*
3 carbohydrates, 1 fat, Freebie vegetables

ROASTED SICILIAN VEGETABLES

PREP TIME: 15 MINUTES
COOK TIME: 30 MINUTES

1 pound medium-size asparagus spears or haricots verts
   (tiny green beans)
2 tablespoons extra virgin olive oil
2 garlic cloves, minced
2 teaspoons chopped fresh thyme
¼ teaspoon salt
¼ teaspoon coarsely ground black pepper
1 pound mixed summer squash (try crookneck and zucchini),
   cut into ½-inch-thick slices
1 cup whole cherry tomatoes
¼ cup pitted kalamata olives

1. Preheat oven to 400°. Coat a jelly roll pan with cooking spray. Wash and trim asparagus; cut into 4-inch spears.

2. Whisk together oil, garlic, thyme, salt, and pepper in a large bowl. Add asparagus and squash; toss to coat. Place drained vegetables on pan and roast 20 minutes, stirring occasionally. Add tomatoes and olives to the same bowl; toss to coat and transfer to baking sheet with asparagus and squash. Arrange in a single layer and roast 10 minutes, stirring occasionally. Serve immediately.

Yield: 8 servings
Serving size: 🍴 *= 1 fat, Freebie vegetables*

SPRING BOUNTY RISOTTO

PREP TIME: 20 MINUTES
COOK TIME: 45 MINUTES

This beautiful side dish is great for entertaining. It also works as a vegetarian entree, thanks to the edamame, a terrific protein source. Arborio rice is short-grain rice that is high in starch and yields a creamy texture when cooked.

3 cups chicken broth (can use lower-sodium version)
2 tablespoons olive oil
½ cup finely chopped onion
½ cup shredded carrots
2 cups Arborio rice (or other short-grain rice)
6 asparagus spears, cut into 1-inch pieces

1 cup diced zucchini
1 cup seeded, diced plum tomatoes
½ cup fresh baby spinach leaves, chopped
½ cup fresh corn kernels
½ cup frozen shelled edamame (green soybeans)
¼ teaspoon freshly ground black pepper
¼ cup finely chopped fresh basil leaves
½ cup grated Parmigiano-Reggiano

1. Bring broth and 3 cups of water to a simmer in a large saucepan. Reduce heat and keep warm.

2. Heat oil in a large heavy saucepan over medium-high heat. Add onion and carrots; sauté 5 minutes, or until vegetables are crisp-tender. Add rice and sauté 2 minutes. Add ½ cup of broth mixture and stir until liquid is nearly absorbed. Add 3 cups of broth mixture and next seven ingredients (asparagus through pepper); cook until liquid is nearly absorbed. Stirring constantly, continue to add broth mixture ½ cup at a time until each addition is absorbed before adding the next. This process will take about 20 minutes until rice is tender and mixture is creamy. (Add additional broth if needed.) Remove from heat; stir in basil and cheese.

Yield: 12 servings

Serving size: ½ 🖐 = 1 protein (fist, ½ fist, or thumb),
2 carbohydrates, 1 fat, Freebie vegetables

WHITE BEAN SOUP IN PUMPERNICKEL BREAD BOWL
SOAK TIME: 6–8 HOURS
PREP TIME: 15 MINUTES
COOK TIME: 1¼ + HOURS

For an added touch, instead of using soup bowls, buy individual bread bowls from a bakery.

1 pound dry white beans, sorted and washed
4 cups chicken broth (can use lower-sodium version)
1 cup chopped onion
¼ cup chopped green pepper
¼ cup chopped red pepper
¼ cup thinly sliced celery
2 garlic cloves, minced
½ teaspoon dried marjoram

(continued on next page)

½ teaspoon dried dill weed
1 teaspoon salt
½ teaspoon red pepper
6 (8-ounce) 5-inch-round individual pumpernickel bread bowls,
*   tops and centers removed (optional)*
¾ cup sliced green onions (optional)

1. Sort, wash, and soak the beans according to package directions. Drain.

2. Add beans to a large stockpot and cover with 3 cups of water and the broth. Add next nine ingredients (onion through red pepper). Bring to a boil, reduce heat, cover, and simmer for 1¼ hours or until beans are tender, stirring occasionally.

3. Ladle soup into bowls or bread bowls in equal-size portions. Garnish each with green onions, if desired.

Yield: 10 servings

Serving size: 🖐 *= 1 protein (fist, ½ fist, or thumb),*
2 carbohydrates (bread not included)

PHENOTYPE D

NO-TIME Recipes

PARMESAN-TOPPED BROCCOLI

PREP TIME: 1 MINUTE
COOK TIME: 5 MINUTES

Tip: To save time, buy broccoli in the produce section that is already washed, cut, bagged, and ready to go.

2 cups fresh broccoli florets
¼ teaspoon salt (optional)
2 tablespoons grated Parmigiano-Reggiano

Combine broccoli, salt, if using, and ¼ cup water in small microwave dish. Cover and cook on high 5 minutes or until broccoli is tender. Drain. Serve topped with cheese.

Yield: 2 servings

Serving size: 🖐 *= 1 protein (fist, ½ fist, or thumb),*
Freebie vegetables

ROASTED MOZZARELLA- AND SPINACH-TOPPED PORTOBELLOS

PREP TIME: 5 MINUTES
COOK TIME: 20 MINUTES

2 portobello mushroom caps
1 garlic clove, minced
¼ teaspoon coarsely ground black pepper
½ cup coarsely chopped fresh spinach
4 ounces fresh mozzarella, sliced
1 tablespoon grated Parmigiano-Reggiano

1. Preheat oven to 400°. Coat foil-lined pan with cooking spray.

2. Wipe mushroom caps gently with damp paper towel. Place on pan; sprinkle with garlic and pepper. Bake 10 minutes; remove. Add spinach and top with mozzarella and Parmesan. Bake an additional 10 minutes; serve warm.

Yield: 2 servings

Serving size: 🍖 *= 2 proteins (fist, ½ fist, or thumb),*
Freebie vegetables

SPICED CARROT-RAISIN SALAD

PREP TIME: 10 MINUTES

Susan's friend Emmy makes this quick salad for potluck dinners because it's a crowd pleaser.

2 (8-ounce) cans crushed pineapple
1 (8-ounce) bag shredded carrots
¼ cup raisins
2 tablespoons chopped fresh parsley
3 tablespoons light mayonnaise
½ teaspoon ground cinnamon
¼ teaspoon ground cumin

Drain pineapple, reserving 1 tablespoon of juice; set aside. Combine pineapple, carrots, raisins, and parsley in a large bowl. Whisk together mayonnaise, reserved juice, and spices; stir into carrot mixture. Cover and refrigerate until ready to serve.

Yield: 4 cups

Serving size: ½ 🌾 *= 1 carbohydrate, Freebie vegetables*

SUSAN'S SUPERQUICK TURKEY CHILI

PREP TIME: 15 MINUTES
COOK TIME: 30 MINUTES

Susan has served this chili for every occasion from New Year's Eve to football games. It's always a hit. She leaves it simmering on the stove and lets people serve themselves. Make a double recipe and freeze the extra for a quick NO-TIME Meal another day.

> 1 tablespoon olive oil
> 1 medium onion, chopped
> 1 small green pepper, chopped
> 1 pound ground turkey breast or soy crumbles
> 2 (10½-ounce) cans condensed tomato soup (can use low-sodium)
> 2 (15-ounce) cans black beans or red kidney beans, drained (rinse to lower
>   sodium more)
> 2 tablespoons chili powder
> ¼ cup shredded reduced-fat Cheddar
> 1 tablespoon sliced green onions (optional)

Heat oil in a large saucepan over medium-high heat; sauté onion and green pepper, about 2 minutes. Add turkey; cook 6 minutes or until browned, stirring to crumble. Stir in soup, beans, and chili powder; bring to a boil. Cover, reduce heat, and simmer 20 minutes, stirring occasionally. Ladle into soup bowls; top with cheese. Garnish with green onions, if desired.

Yield: 5 servings

Serving size: 🏈 *= 1 protein, 3 carbohydrates, 1 fat*

MORE-TIME Recipes

EASY ONION CHICKEN

Cathy's mother-in-law makes this family favorite whenever the Christie clan gathers.

PREP TIME: 10 MINUTES
COOK TIME: 55 MINUTES

> 6 tablespoons flour
> ½ teaspoon paprika
> ¼ teaspoon coarsely ground black pepper
> 6 5-ounce skinless chicken breast halves

2 tablespoons olive oil
1 (1.3-ounce) envelope Lipton dry onion soup mix

1. Sift together flour, paprika, and pepper. Dredge chicken in flour mixture.

2. Heat oil in a large Dutch oven over medium-high heat; add chicken and brown on both sides, about 5 minutes. Add soup mix and enough water to cover. Bring to a boil, reduce heat, and cover. Simmer 45 minutes, or until chicken is tender.

Yield: 6 servings

Serving size: 🐟 *= 1 protein and 1 fat*

LENTIL-VEGETABLE SOUP

PREP TIME: 15 MINUTES
COOK TIME: 40 MINUTES

2 cups dry lentils
7 cups low-sodium chicken broth
4 celery stalks, chopped
3 medium carrots, shredded
2 medium onions, chopped
2 small potatoes, diced
3 garlic cloves, minced
3 parsley sprigs, chopped
2 tablespoons fresh basil (or 1 teaspoon dried basil)
1 teaspoon cayenne pepper
1 bay leaf
*1 (28-ounce) can chopped tomatoes with liquid (can use lower-sodium
    version)*

Combine lentils and broth in a large Dutch oven; bring to boil. Cover, reduce heat, and simmer 20 minutes. Add next nine ingredients (celery through bay leaf); cover and simmer 10 minutes. Add tomatoes; cook an additional 10 minutes. Discard bay leaf.

Yield: 10 servings

Serving size: 🥄 *= 1 protein (fist, ½ fist, or thumb), 2 carbohydrates,*
Freebie *vegetables*

PHENOTYPE E

NO-TIME Recipes

NUTTY-FRUITY SPINACH SALAD WITH ORANGE DRESSING
PREP TIME: 5 MINUTES

> *4 cups baby spinach leaves*
> *½ cup diced apples (such as Granny Smith or Gala)*
> *1 green onion, sliced*
> *¼ cup golden raisins*
> *¼ cup coarsely chopped walnuts*

Place spinach on large platter. Arrange apples, onion, raisins, and walnuts on spinach; drizzle with Orange Dressing.

Yield: 5 cups

Serving size: 👊 *= 1 protein (fist, ½ fist, or thumb),*
1 carbohydrate, plus 1 fat for dressing (see below);
Freebie *vegetables*

Orange Dressing
PREP TIME: 5 MINUTES

> *1 cup cider vinegar*
> *2 heaping tablespoons orange marmalade*
> *½ cup sugar (can use sugar substitute)*
> *2 teaspoons dry mustard*
> *2 teaspoons salt (optional or can use less)*
> *½ teaspoon freshly ground black pepper*
> *½ teaspoon hot sauce*
> *⅔ cup canola oil*

Combine first seven ingredients (vinegar through hot sauce) in a blender; process until smooth. Slowly add oil through feed tube, processing until blended.

Yield: 32 servings

Serving size: 🥄 *= 1 fat*

MEDITERRANEAN PASTA WITH SUN-DRIED TOMATOES AND FETA

PREP TIME: 10 MINUTES
COOK TIME: 9–11 MINUTES

During a trip to California, Susan's friend Tandy made this pasta dish. Susan begged her for the recipe because it's so easy, colorful, and fun.

Tip: To roast garlic, cut top from garlic head and place on a 6 x 6-inch foil square; drizzle with olive oil. Loosely close foil around garlic and seal. Roast at 350° for 1 hour; cool 5 minutes.

6 ounces uncooked whole wheat linguine
1 whole garlic head, roasted and mashed
4 sun-dried tomatoes packed in oil, cut into strips
½ (4-ounce) package crumbled feta cheese
½ cup finely chopped parsley
¼ cup pine nuts, toasted
¼ cup sliced black olives
¼ teaspoon salt

Cook pasta according to package directions; drain. Combine pasta and remaining ingredients in a large bowl; toss gently.

Yield: 2 servings
Serving size: 1½ 🍴 = 1 protein, 3 carbohydrates, 1 fat

PHYTO-FRUIT SMOOTHIE: LIME-ONADE

PREP TIME: 5 MINUTES

1 banana
½ cup low-fat vanilla frozen yogurt
½ cup lemon or lime sherbet
2 tablespoons limeade concentrate
2 teaspoons lemon juice
2 teaspoons honey

Place all ingredients into a blender or food processor. Blend thoroughly.

Yield: approximately 2 servings
Serving size: 🍴 = 3 carbohydrates

SO EASY CAESAR SALAD

PREP TIME: 10 MINUTES

> 1 small head romaine lettuce
> 2 tablespoons grated Parmigiano-Reggiano
> 2 tablespoons light Caesar dressing
> 1 slice sourdough or Italian bread, toasted and cubed (optional or can use
>   a whole grain bread)
> 2 anchovies (optional)

Wash and dry lettuce; cut into bite-sized pieces. Place in salad bowl with cheese and dressing; toss. Garnish with croutons and anchovies, if desired.

Yield: 2 servings

Serving size: 1½ 🏈 = 1 protein (fist, ½ fist, or thumb),
1 fat, Freebie vegetables

MORE-TIME Recipes

COMFORT-STYLE CHICKEN SOUP

PREP TIME: 15 MINUTES
COOK TIME: 50 MINUTES

Our friend Marlene makes this updated version of everyone's favorite soup in the fall and brings it to the office to share.

> 2 tablespoons canola oil
> 1 pound skinless, boneless chicken breasts, coarsely chopped
> 2 large carrots, thinly sliced
> 1 large onion, diced
> 1 celery stalk, sliced
> ½ teaspoon salt
> ¼ teaspoon coarsely ground black pepper
> ½ teaspoon celery seeds (optional)
> ½ teaspoon dried rosemary, crushed (optional)
> 4 cups chicken broth (can use lower-sodium version)
> 2 large potatoes, diced
> 5 fresh rosemary sprigs (optional)

1. Heat 1 tablespoon of the oil in a large Dutch oven over medium-high heat. Add chicken; cook until browned, stirring occasionally. Remove and set aside.

2. Sauté carrots, onion, celery, salt, and pepper in remaining tablespoon of oil for 2 minutes. Add celery seeds and rosemary; cook for 1 minute. Add broth, 4 cups of water, and potatoes; bring to boil, reduce heat, and simmer 30 minutes. Add chicken to soup mixture, cook 10 minutes. Ladle into bowls and garnish with rosemary, if desired.

Yield: 8 servings

Serving size: 🖐 *= 1 protein, 2 carbohydrates, 1 fat, Freebie vegetables*

CRAB CAKES NEW ORLEANS

PREP TIME: 20 MINUTES
COOK TIME: 30 MINUTES

Casually elegant and perfect for a cozy dinner party.

  1 tablespoon canola oil
  2 garlic cloves, minced
  2 tablespoons finely chopped onions
  2 tablespoons finely sliced green onions
  2 tablespoons finely chopped fresh parsley
  ½ cup dry bread crumbs
  1 tablespoon Dijon mustard
  1 tablespoon Worcestershire sauce
  ¼ teaspoon salt (optional)
  ¼ teaspoon red pepper
  ¼ teaspoon white pepper
  ½ pound lump crabmeat, picked for shells
  1 whole egg
  1 egg white

1. Preheat oven to 375°. Coat foil-lined baking sheet with cooking spray.

2. Heat oil in small nonstick skillet over medium-high heat; sauté garlic, onions, green onions, and parsley for 2 minutes. Remove from heat; transfer to a large mixing bowl. Add next six ingredients (bread crumbs through white pepper) to onion mixture. Add crabmeat, egg, and egg white; combine thoroughly. Shape into 4 crab cakes and place on prepared baking sheet. If you prefer, you can also cook the cakes in a skillet.

3. Bake 15 minutes. Carefully turn crab cakes; bake an additional 15 minutes or until golden brown. Served plain, with mustard, or marinara sauce.

Yield: 4 servings

Serving size: 🐟 *= 1 protein, 1 carbohydrate, 1 fat*

ROMAN-STYLE CHICKEN CACCIATORE

PREP TIME: 15 MINUTES
COOK TIME: 40 MINUTES

1 tablespoon olive oil
4 skinless, boneless chicken breast halves, 4 to 6 ounces each
¾ teaspoon salt
¼ cup chopped onion
1 garlic clove, minced
¾ cup sliced fresh mushrooms
½ (14½-ounce) can chopped tomatoes with liquid (can use lower sodium
  version)
½ cup chopped green pepper
3 tablespoons dry red wine
½ teaspoon dried oregano
¼ teaspoon coarsely ground black pepper
½ teaspoon paprika
2 teaspoons cornstarch
4 fresh mushroom caps

1. Heat 1½ teaspoons of the oil in a large nonstick skillet over medium-high heat. Add chicken and sprinkle with ¼ teaspoon salt; sauté for 2 minutes on each side or until lightly browned. Remove chicken and set aside.

2. Heat the remaining 1½ teaspoons oil in skillet; sauté onion and garlic 3 minutes. Stir in mushrooms, tomatoes, green pepper, wine, oregano, remaining ½ teaspoon salt, and pepper. Return chicken to skillet and bring to a boil. Cover, reduce heat, and simmer for 25 minutes, or until chicken is done. Transfer to serving platter, sprinkle with paprika, and keep warm.

3. Combine cornstarch with 2 tablespoons cold water and stir into vegetable mixture; add mushroom caps. Cook and stir until sauce is thick and bubbly, 1 minute. Spoon sauce over chicken and top each serving with a mushroom cap.

Yield: 4 servings

Serving size: 🥄 *1 protein, 1 fat, Freebie vegetables*

PHENOTYPE H

NO-TIME Recipes

PHYTO-FRUIT SMOOTHIE: PIÑA COOLADA

PREP TIME: 5 MINUTES

1 banana
1 cup low-fat vanilla frozen yogurt
½ cup pineapple juice
¼ cup shredded coconut

Place all ingredients into a blender or food processor. Blend thoroughly.

Yield: approximately 2 servings

Serving size: 🍸 *= 1 protein, 2 carbohydrates, 1 fat*

PHYTO-FRUIT SMOOTHIE: SHIP A-SOY

PREP TIME: 5 MINUTES

1 banana
1 cup low-fat vanilla frozen yogurt
½ cup low-fat soy milk
3–4 tablespoons frozen orange juice concentrate
2 tablespoons wheat germ

Place all ingredients into a blender or food processor. Blend thoroughly.

Yield: approximately 2 servings

Serving size: 🍸 *= 1 protein, 2 carbohydrates*

MORE-TIME Recipes

GOOD LUCK HOPPIN' JOHN

SOAK TIME: 12 HOURS
PREP TIME: 15 MINUTES
COOK TIME: 1–1¼ HOURS

Black-eyed peas are a New Year's Day tradition for many families in the South because they are thought to bring good luck.

(continued on next page)

1 pound dry black-eyed peas
1 cup brown rice
1 tablespoon olive or canola oil
1 large onion, finely chopped
6 cups chicken broth (can use lower sodium version)
1½ teaspoon dried oregano
1 teaspoon garlic salt
½ cup sliced green onions

1. Soak peas according to package directions; drain. Prepare rice according to package direction while beans are cooking. Keep warm.

2. Heat oil in a large Dutch oven over medium-high heat. Sauté onion about 3 minutes; add peas, chicken broth, oregano, and garlic salt. Bring to boil; reduce heat, cover, and simmer 1–1¼ hours, or until peas are tender. Serve over rice; garnish with green onions.

Yield: 8 servings

Serving size: 🍴 *= 1 protein (fist, ½ fist, or thumb), 1 carbohydrate*

HERB-RUBBED PORK TENDERLOIN WITH ALMOND-APRICOT ORZO

Prep time: 10 minutes
Cook time: 35 minutes
Resting time: 10 minutes

You can also serve the pork tenderloin with the Wild Mushroom Risotto. It's a tasty combination too.

2 garlic cloves, minced
2 tablespoons minced onion
2 tablespoons chopped fresh parsley
2 tablespoons chopped fresh sage
½ teaspoon salt
¼ teaspoon coarsely ground black pepper
1 pork tenderloin, trimmed (approximately 12 ounces)

1. Preheat oven to 375°. Coat a 13 x 9-inch baking dish with cooking spray.

2. Combine garlic, onion, parsley, sage, salt, and pepper; rub over pork. Place in baking dish. Roast uncovered, 30 to 35 minutes, or until thermometer reads 160° (slightly pink). Remove from oven, cover, and let

stand 10 minutes before slicing. Slice on diagonal and serve with Almond-Apricot Orzo.

Yield: 3 servings

Serving size: 🍖 *= 1 protein plus 3 carbohydrates and 1 fat for orzo (see below)*

Almond-Apricot Orzo

PREP TIME: 5 MINUTES
COOK TIME: 15 MINUTES

1 cup orzo (rice-shaped pasta)
2 tablespoons golden raisins
¼ cup dried apricots, cut into strips
1½ teaspoon canola oil
¼ cup finely chopped almonds
1 tablespoon honey

1. Prepare orzo according to package directions; drain and transfer to large bowl. Plump raisins and apricots in hot water for 1 minute; drain.

2. Heat oil in a nonstick medium skillet over medium heat; sauté almonds until lightly browned. Add raisins and apricots; cook 4 minutes to blend flavors, stirring occasionally. Add sautéed mixture and honey to orzo; toss gently.

Yield: 5 servings

Serving size: ½ 🏈 *= 3 carbohydrates, 1 fat*

TAILGATE CHILI

PREP TIME: 20 MINUTES
COOK TIME: 1–1½ HOURS

This recipe makes a large amount, perfect for a tailgate party before the big game.

2 tablespoons olive oil
1½ pounds skinless, boneless chicken breast, cubed
½ teaspoon ground black pepper
1 large onion, chopped
3 garlic cloves, minced

(continued on next page)

    2 (15.8-ounce) cans black-eyed peas, drained (rinse to lower sodium even more)

    1 (15.8-ounce) can Great Northern beans, drained (rinse to lower sodium even more)

    5 cups chicken broth (can use lower-sodium version)

    1 (14½-ounce) can stewed tomatoes (can use lower-sodium version)

    1 (12-ounce) bottle beer

    2 (4½-ounce) cans chopped green chilies

    ½ teaspoon dried oregano

    ½ teaspoon ground cumin

    ¼ teaspoon lemon pepper

    2 cups reduced-fat shredded Monterey Jack cheese

    2 cups salsa (optional)

    1 cup reduced-fat sour cream (optional)

1. Heat 1 tablespoon of the oil in a large Dutch oven over medium-high heat. Season chicken with pepper and brown in Dutch oven; remove and set aside.

2. Heat remaining oil in the same Dutch oven over medium-high heat. Add onion and garlic; sauté 5 minutes. Return chicken to Dutch oven; add black-eyed peas and next eight ingredients (Great Northern beans through lemon pepper). Add 1 cup cheese. Bring to a boil; cover, reduce heat, and simmer 1–1½ hours. Serve garnished with cheese, salsa, or sour cream.

Yield: 16 servings

Serving size: 🍴 *= 1 protein, 2 carbohydrates, 1 fat*

WILD MUSHROOM RISOTTO

PREP TIME: 15 MINUTES
COOK TIME: 30 MINUTES

If you like mushrooms, you will love this recipe. It has a very "earthy" flavor.

    2 tablespoons olive oil

    1 cup chopped shallots or green onions

    2 large garlic cloves, minced

    1 pound fresh mixed mushrooms (such as shiitake and crimini), sliced

    2 tablespoons chopped fresh thyme (or 2 teaspoons dried)

    ¼ teaspoon salt

    ¼ teaspoon coarsely ground black pepper

    1½ cups Arborio rice (or other short-grain rice)

    ½ cup dry white wine

3½ to 4 cups chicken broth (can use lower sodium version)
2 cups baby spinach leaves
⅓ cup freshly grated Parmigiano-Reggiano (about 1 ounce)

1. Heat 1 tablespoon of oil in a large nonstick saucepan over medium-high heat; sauté shallots and garlic about 2 minutes. Add mushrooms, thyme, salt, and pepper; sauté until juices evaporate, about 5 minutes.

2. Add rice and remaining tablespoon of oil, stirring to coat; sauté 2 minutes. Add wine; cook 2 minutes or until liquid is nearly absorbed, stirring constantly. Add broth, ½ cup at a time, until each addition is absorbed before adding the next. Stir constantly, 20 minutes or longer, until rice is tender and mixture is creamy. (Add additional broth if risotto becomes dry.) Add spinach and stir until wilted. Remove from heat; stir in cheese.

Yield: 16 servings

Serving size: ½ *= 1 carbohydrate,* Freebie *vegetables*

Antioxidant-Rich Foods

TOP TWENTY ANTIOXIDANT FOODS

Asparagus	Citrus
Blueberries	Winter squash
Broccoli	Green, red, and orange peppers
Cantaloupe	Strawberries
Carrots	Leafy greens
Nectarines	Watermelon
Papaya	Beets
Peaches	Mangoes
Spinach	Pumpkin
Tomatoes	Cabbage

WAYS TO ADD ANTIOXIDANTS

Instead of:	Use:
Iceberg lettuce	Romaine, spinach, red leaf, or mesclun salad mix
Tomato sauce	Vegetable sauce (add shredded carrots or zucchini, see recipe for Vegetable Spaghetti Sauce in Appendix C, Phenotype C)
Cole slaw	Cabbage and broccoslaw (bagged in the produce section)
White potatoes	Sweet potatoes

Fat Comparison

What's the big deal about substituting monounsaturated fats for saturated fats and trans fats?

There's no doubt that a steady diet of saturated and hydrogenated fat ratchets up the blood LDL levels. In fact, the Institute of Medicine (IOM) stated in a public briefing that the maximum safe intake for saturated fat and trans fat is *zero*. Realizing that extreme changes would be needed to totally eliminate all these fats, and that some saturated fats are worse than others, you want to set a goal of reducing your consumption of trans fats and saturated fat as much as possible.

How do you track them down and reduce or remove them from your diet? Saturated fats are found in animal food products such as fatty meat, whole milk, butter, lard, and cheese. Trans fats or hydrogenated fats are in almost every processed, baked, and fried food and most margarine. Look closely at the ingredient label. The words "partially hydrogenated oil," regardless of whether the oil is soybean, corn, or any other, mean the same thing as trans fat. Hydrogenated fats and trans fats have the same negative effect in your body as saturated fats.

PARTIALLY HYDROGENATED OIL = TRANS FAT and has the same negative effect in your body as saturated fat.

Major Food Sources of Saturated Fat

Fatty meats, bacon, sausage; full-fat dairy products such as whole milk, cream, sour cream, cheese, and butter; lard; bakery products; coconut oil, palm oil, palm kernel oil

Major Food Sources of Trans (Partially Hydrogenated) Fat

Baked goods such as doughnuts, cookies, breads, cakes, and crackers; almost any shelf-stable processed item that includes fat (look on the label for "partially hydrogenated" as one of the first three ingredients); margarines with partially hydrogenated fat as the first ingredient; French fries, restaurant or takeout

Major Food Sources of Nonhydrogenated Unsaturated Fat—Use instead of fats above

Olive oil, canola oil, avocado, nuts and seeds, olives, walnut oil, grapeseed oil, hazelnut oil, corn oil, soybean oil, peanut oil, pumpkin oil, sesame oil; although only olive oil and canola oil are listed as Focus Foods, any of these nonhydrogenated unsaturated fats can be used

High-Fiber Foods

High-Fiber Food Selections		Amount of Fiber (Grams)
Kidney beans, 1 cup canned		16.4
Black beans, 1 cup cooked		15.0
Lima beans, 1 cup cooked		13.2
Garbanzos, 1 cup canned		12.5
Raspberries, 1 cup frozen		11.0
All-Bran cereal, ½ cup	½	9.6
Peas, split, ½ cup cooked	½	8.1
Raspberries, 1 cup raw		8.0
Lentils, ½ cup cooked	½	7.8
Prunes, 1 cup		7.7
Raisin bran, 1 cup		7.5
Artichoke, 1 medium cooked		6.5
Winter squash, 1 cup baked		5.7
Turnip greens, 1 cup boiled and drained		5.6
Broccoli, 1 cup frozen cooked		5.5

(continued on next page)

High-Fiber Food Selections			Amount of Fiber (Grams)
Pear, 1 medium fresh			5.1
Shredded wheat, 1 cup			5.0
Carrots, 1 cup cooked			4.7
Figs, 2, dried			4.6
Beans, ½ cup canned			4.5
Green beans, 1 cup cooked			4.0
Strawberries, 1 cup sliced frozen			3.8
Apple (with skin), 1			3.7
Peas, green, ½ cup canned			3.5
Brown rice, 1 cup cooked			3.5
Cauliflower, 1 cup cooked			3.3
Strawberries, 1 cup sliced raw			3.3
Orange, 1			3.1
Sunflower seed kernels, ¼ cup dry roasted			2.9
Banana, 1			2.8
Oat bran muffin, 1 medium			2.6
Cheerios, 1 cup			2.6
Oatmeal, cooked			2.0

Source: USDA Nutrient Database (see Resource List for Web site).

Caffeine Content in Various Beverages

Beverages	Serving Size	Caffeine (Milligrams)	
		AVERAGE	RANGE
Canned iced tea	1 cup (8 oz.)	17	10–24
Chocolate milk	1 cup (8 oz.)	5	2–7
Coffee, drip	1 cup (8 oz.)	184	176–240
Coffee, instant	1 cup (8 oz.)	104	65–120
Coffee, decaf	1 cup (8 oz.)	5	3–8
Coffee, espresso	¼ cup (2 oz.)	100	80–120
Cola soft drink	1 cup (8 oz.)	30	29–39
Hot chocolate	1 cup (8 oz.)	6	3–32
Tea, brewed, U.S. brand	1 cup (8 oz.)	47	32–144
Tea, brewed, imported	1 cup (8 oz.)	60	40–176
Tea, green	1 cup (8 oz.)	15	10–25
Tea, instant	1 cup (8 oz.)	30	20–50

Mercury Content in
Fish and Seafood

Do you need to be concerned about mercury poisoning and the level of mercury in fish? If you are a woman of childbearing age or pregnant, and eating fish regularly, the answer may be *yes*. Although the risk–benefit ratio currently seems to indicate more benefit than risk, eating a *variety* of fish is the best policy.

LOWER-MERCURY FISH AND SEAFOOD

- Shrimp
- Clams
- Scallops
- Lobster
- Trout
- Catfish
- Cod and flounder
- Salmon and canned tuna

HIGHER-MERCURY FISH

- Tuna steak
- Swordfish
- Tilefish
- King mackerel

Resources

Company/Product	Web Site/E-mail/Address	Phone Number
Accusplit	www.accusplit.com	800-935-1996
Amy's Organic Frozen Dinners	www.amys.com amy@amyskitchen.net	707-578-7188
Benecol Light	www.benecol.com	888-BENECOL
Cabot Creamery	www.cabotcheese.com Cabot Creamery 1 Home Farm Way Montpelier, VT 05602	800-762-2268
Cheerios	www.cheerios.com	800-328-1144
The Cherry Stop Dried cherries	www.cherrystop.com	800-286-7209
Chocolat Debauve Gallais	www.debauve-et-gallais.com info@debauve-et-gallais.com 30 Rue des Saints-Perès Paris VII, France	33-1-45-48-54-67

(continued on next page)

Company/Product	Web Site/E-mail/Address	Phone Number

Clif Bar
  Chocolate Chip Peanut
  Crunch
	www.clifbar.com	800-884-5254

ConsumerLab.com, LLC	www.consumerlab.com	914-722-9149
New Lifestyles, Inc. Digi-Walker	www.digiwalker.com	816-353-1721
Eggland's Best Eggs	www.eggland.com	800-922-EGGS
Emeril's Seasonings	www.emerils.com Emeril's Homebase Merchandise Sales 829 St. Charles Ave. New Orleans, LA 70130	
Evian Mineral Water	www.evian.com	800-633-3363
GeniSoy Soy Nuts	www.genisoy.com	800-GENISOY
Harry and David's Honey & Dill Mustard	www.harryanddavid.com	

Hodgson Mill
  Multi Grain Hot Cereal with
  Flaxseed and Soy
	www.hodgsonmill.com	800-347-0105

Ken's Lite Dressings
  Raspberry Walnut Vinaigrette
  Vidalia Onion Dressing
	www.kensfoods.com
	Ken's Foods, Inc.
	Marlborough, MA 01752
		800-645-5707

Laughing Cow Cheese	Bel/Kaukauna, Inc. P. O. Box 1974 Kaukauna, WI 54130	800-993-8625
Lean Cuisine Jumbo Rigatoni	www.nestleusa.com www.leancuisine.com	
McCann's Irish steel-cut oatmeal	www.mccanns.ie	201-934-6953

Morningstar Farms
  Soy Burger—Black Bean
  Soy Sausage
	www.morningstarfarms.com	800-557-6525

Newman's Own Salad Dressing Balsamic Vinaigrette	www.newmansown.com	

COMPANY/PRODUCT	WEB SITE/E-MAIL/ADDRESS	PHONE NUMBER
Odwalla Bar Peanut Crunch	www.odwalla.com	800-odwalla
Olivio Premium Products Margarine, low in trans fat	www.olivioproducts.com	
Perrier Mineral Water	www.minere.com/perrier.htm	
Powerbar Harvest Peanut Butter Chocolate Chip	www.powerbar.com	800-58-POWER
Quaker Oat Squares	www.quakeroats.com	312-821-1000
Rosemount Estate Wines	www.rosemountestates.com	800-255-9966
San Pellegrino Sparkling Natural Mineral Water	www.sanpellegrino.com	800-255-8334
Sargento Reduced fat Mexican Cheese	www.sargentocheese.com	800-CHEESES (800-243-3737)
Seeds of Change	www.seedsofchange.co.uk	
Smart Balance	www.smartbalance.com	
Stonyfield's Organic Yogurt Banilla low-fat yogurt	www.stonyfield.com	800-PRO-COWS
SupplementWatch, Inc.	www.supplementwatch.com	801-712-0408
Take Control	www.takecontrol.com	800-259-4835
Triscuits	www.kraftfoods.com	
Vermont maple syrup	www.madeinvermont.com	877-471-7308
McNeil Nutritionals Viactiv Soft Calcium Chews	www.viactiv.com	877-VIACTIV
Vittel Mineral Water	www.minere.com/vittel.htm	
USDA National Nutrient Database	www.nal.usda.gov/fnic/cgi-bin/ nut_search.pl	

Williams Sonoma
   Olio Santo Blood Orange
     Olive Oil
   Olio Santo Eureka Lemon
     Olive Oil
	www.williams-sonoma.com
	Williams-Sonoma, Inc.
	San Francisco, CA 94109
		877-812-6235

References

CHAPTER 1: OUTSMARTING YOUR GENETIC LEGACY

Coulston, A. M., M. J. Feeney, and L. Hoolihan. The challenge to customize. *Journal of the American Dietetic Association* 103, no. 4 (2003): 443–44.

Cousins, R. J. Nutritional regulation of gene expression. *The American Journal of Medicine* 106, no. 1A (1999): 20S–23S.

Dauncey, M. J., P. White, K. A. Burton, and M. Katsumata. Nutrition-hormone receptor-gene interactions: Implications for development and disease. *Proceedings of the Nutrition Society* 60, no. 1 (2001): 63–72.

Fogg-Johnson, N., and J. Kaput. Nutrigenomics: An emerging scientific discipline. The identification and understanding of individual and population differences and similarities in gene expression in response to diet can lead to food products customized for an individual's nutritional needs. *Food Technology* 57, no. 4 (2003): 60–67.

Venter, J. C., et al. The sequence of the human genome. *Science* 291 (2001): 1304–51.

Willett, W. C. Balancing lifestyle and genomics research for disease prevention. *Science* 296 (2002): 695–98.

CHAPTER 2: LEARN YOUR PHENOTYPE AND WHAT TRIGGERS YOUR WEIGHT GAIN

Coulson, A. S., et al. RAGs: A novel approach to computerized genetic risk assessment and decision support from pedigrees. *Methods Information in Medicine* 40, no. 4 (2001): 315–22.

Gilpin, C. A., et al. A preliminary validation of family history assessment form to select women at risk for breast or ovarian cancer for referral to a genetics center. *Clinical Genetics* 58, no. 4 (2000): 299–308.

Higgins, M., et al. NHLBI family heart study: Objectives and design. *American Journal of Epidemiology* 143 (1996): 1219–28.

Hunt, S. C., et al. A comparison of positive family history definitions for defining risk of future disease. *Journal of Chronic Diseases* 39, no. 10 (1986): 809–21.

Janssen, I., A. Fortier, R. Hudson, and R. Ross. Effects of an energy-restrictive diet with or without exercise on abdominal fat, intramuscular fat, and metabolic risk factors in obese women. *Diabetes Care* 25, no. 3 (2002): 431–38.

Ma, Y., E. R. Bertone, E. J. Stanek III, G. W. Reed, J. R. Hebert, N. L. Cohen, P. A. Merriam, and I. S. Ockene. Association between eating patterns and obesity in a free-living U.S. adult population. *American Journal of Epidemiology* 158 (2003): 85–92.

Ponder, M., et al. Family history and perceived vulnerability to some common diseases: A study of young people and their parents. *Journal of Medical Genetics* 33 (1996): 485–92.

Ross, R. Effects of diet and exercise induced weight loss on visceral adipose tissue in men and women. *Sports Medicine* 24, no. 1 (1997): 55–64.

Ross, R., and I. Janssen. Is abdominal fat preferentially reduced in response to exercise-induced weight loss? *Medicine and Science in Sports and Exercise* 31, suppl. no. 11 (1999): S568–S572.

Ross, R., H. Pedwell, and J. Rissanen. Response of total and regional lean tissue and skeletal muscle to a program of energy restriction and resistance exercise. *International Journal of Obesity and Related Metabolic Disorders* 19, no. 11 (1995): 781–87.

Ross, R., J. Rissanen, H. Pedwell, J. Clifford, and P. Shragge. Study School of Physical Education, Queens University, Kingston, Ontario Canada. Influence of diet and exercise on skeletal muscle and visceral adipose tissue in men. *Journal of Applied Physiology* 81, no. 6 (1996): 2445–55.

Silberberg, J., et al. Comparison of family history measures used to identify high risk of coronary heath disease. *Genetic Epidemiology* 16 (1999): 344–55.

Stunkard, A. J., and S. Messick. The three-factor eating questionnaire to measure dietary restraint, disinhibition and hunger. *Journal of Psychosomatic Research* 29, no. 1 (1985): 71–83.

Williams, R. R., et al. Health family trees: A tool for finding and helping young family members of coronary and cancer prone pedigrees in Texas and Utah. *American Journal of Public Health* 78, no. 10 (1988): 1283–86.

Williams, R. R., et al. Usefulness of cardiovascular family history data for population-based preventive medicine and medical research (The Health Family Tree Study and the NHLBI Family Heart Study). *The American Journal of Cardiology* 87 (2001) 129–35.

Yoon, P. W., et al. Can family history be used as a tool for public health and preventive medicine? *Genetics in Medicine* 4, no. 4 (2002): 304–10.

CHAPTER 4: THE PHENOTYPE A DIET

Anton, R. F., and D. J. Drobes. Clinical measurement of craving in addiction. *Psychiatric Annals* 28, no. 10 (1998): 553.

Berg, F. *Women Afraid to Eat.* Hettinger, N.Dak.: Healthy Weight Network, 2000.

Blum, K., et al. Dopamine D2 receptor gene variants: Association and linkage studies in impulsive-addictive compulsive behavior. *Pharmacogenetics* 5, no. 3 (1995): 121–41.

Blum, K., et al. Reward deficiency syndrome. *American Scientist* 84, no. 2 (1996): 132–45.

Bruce, B., and D. Wilfrey. Binge eating among the overweight population: A serious and prevalent problem. *Journal of the American Dietetic Association* 96, no. 1 (1996): 58.

Bulik, C. M., P. F. Sullivan, and K. S. Kendler. Medical and psychiatric morbidity in obese women with and without binge eating. *International Journal of Eating Disorders* 32, no. 1 (2002): 72–78.

Cohen, J. H., A. R. Kristal, D. Neumark-Sztainer, C. L. Rock, and M. L. Neuhouser. Psychological distress is associated with unhealthful dietary practices. *Journal of the American Dietetic Association* 102, no. 5 (2002): 699–703.

Drewnowski, A., and A. S. Levine. Sugar and fat—from genes to culture. *The Journal of Nutrition* 133, no. 3 (2003): S829–S830.

Fairburn, C. G., and G. T. Wilson. *Binge Eating—Nature, Assessment, and Treatment.* New York: Guilford Press, 1993.

Fairburn, C. G., H. A. Doll, S. L. Welch, P. J. Hay, et al. Risk factors for binge-eating disorder: A community-based case-control study. *Archives of General Psychiatry* 55, no. 5 (1998): 425.

Fassino, S., P. Leombruni, A. Piero, G. Abbate-Daga, and G. Giacomo Rovera. Mood, eating attitudes, and anger in obese women with and without binge-eating disorder. *Journal of Psychosomatic Research* 54, no. 6 (2003): 559–66.

Fitzgibbon, M. I., L. A. Sanchez-Johnson, and Z. Martinovich. A test of the continuity perspective across bulimic and binge-eating pathology. *International Journal of Eating Disorders* 34, no. 1 (2003): 83–97.

Grilo, C. M., R. M. Masheb, and G. T. Wilson. Subtyping binge-eating disorder. *Journal of Consulting and Clinical Psychology* 69, no. 6 (2001): 1066–72.

Kalman, D., H. Cascarano, D. R. Krieger, T. Incledon, and M. Woolsey. Frequency of binge-eating disorder in an outpatient weight loss clinic. *Journal of the American Dietetic Association* 102, no. 5 (2002): 697–99.

Kensinger, G. J., M. A. Murtaugh, S. K. Reichman, and C. C. Tangney. Psychological symptoms are greater among weight cycling women with severe binge-eating behavior. *Journal of the American Dietetic Association* 98, no. 8 (1998): 863–68.

Neumark-Sztainer, D., R. Butler, and H. Palti. Dieting and binge-eating: Which dieters are at risk? *Journal of the American Dietetic Association* 95, no. 5 (1995): 586.

Pelchat, M. L. Of human bondage: Food craving, obsession, compulsion, and addiction. *Physiology & Behavior* 76, no. 3 (2002): 347–52.

Pinaquy, S., H. Chabrol, C. Simon, J. P. Louvet, and P. Barbe. Emotional eating, alexithymia, and binge-eating disorder in obese women. *Obesity Research* 11, no. 2 (2003): 195–201.

Reeves, R. S., R. S. McPherson, M. Z. Nichaman, R. B. Harrist, et al. Nutrient intake of obese female binge eaters. *Journal of the American Dietetic Association* 101, no. 2 (2001): 209–15.

Tuschen-Caffier, B., and C. Vogele. Psychological and physiological reactivity to stress: An experimental study on bulimic patients, restrained eaters and controls. *Psychotherapy and Psychometrics* 68, no. 6 (1999): 333.

Wang, G., N. D. Volkow, J. Logan, N. R. Pappas, et al. Brain dopamine and obesity. *The Lancet* 357, no. 9253 (2001): 354–57.

Weinberg, B. A., and B. K. Bealer. *The Caffeine Advantage.* New York: Free Press, 2002.

Yanovski, S. Sugar and fat: Cravings and aversions. *The Journal of Nutrition* 133, no. 3 (2003): S835–S837.

CHAPTER 5: THE PHENOTYPE B DIET

American Dietetic Association. Health implications of dietary fiber. *Journal of the American Dietetic Association* 102, no. 7 (2002): 993–1000.

Beitz, R., G. B. M. Mensink, and B. Fischer. Blood pressure and vitamin C and fruit and vegetable intake. *Annals of Nutrition & Metabolism* 47, no. 5 (2003): 214–20.

Benedetti, R. G., K. J. Wise, and L. K. Massey. The hemodynamic effect of dietary calcium supplementation on rat renovascular hypertension. *Basic Research in Cardiology* 88, no. 1 (1993): 60–71.

Braschi, A., D. J. Naismith, and A. Braschi. The effect of low-dose potassium supplementation on blood pressure in apparently healthy volunteers. *British Journal of Nutrition* 90, no. 1 (2003): 53–60.

Caulfield, M., et al. Genome-wide mapping of human loci for essential hypertension. *The Lancet* 361, no. 9375 (2003): 2118–123.

DASH Eating Plan. National Institutes of Health, National Heart, Lung, and Blood Institute, U.S. Department of Health and Human Services, 2003.

Dekkers, J. C., F. A. Treiber, G. Kapuku, and H. Sneider. Differential influence of family history of hypertension and premature myocardial infarction on systolic blood pressure and left ventricular mass trajectories in youth. *Pediatrics* 111, no. 6 (2003): 1387–93.

Dominiczak, A. F., D. C. Negrin, J. S. Clark, and M. J. Brosnan. Genes and hypertension: from gene mapping in experimental models to vascular gene transfer strategies. *Hypertension* 35, no. 1 (2000): 164.

Faria, A. N., F. F. R. Filho, S. R. G. Ferreira, and M. T. Zanella. Impact of visceral fat on blood pressure and insulin sensitivity in hypertensive obese women. *Obesity Research* 10 (2002): 1203–6.

Harrap, S. B. Where are all the blood-pressure genes? *The Lancet* 361, no. 9375 (2003): 2149–51.

Hunter, D. J., et al. Genetic contribution to renal function and electrolyte balance: a twin study. *Clinical Science* 103, no. 3 (2002): 259–65.

Karanja, N. M., M. L. McCullough, S. K. Kumanyika, K. L. Pedula, et al. Preenrollment diets of Dietary Approaches to Stop Hypertension trial participants. *Journal of the American Dietetic Association* 99, suppl. no. 8 (1999): S28–S34.

Kwok, T. C., T. Y. Chan, and J. Woo. Relationship of urinary sodium/potassium excretion and calcium intake to blood pressure and prevalence of hypertension among older Chinese vegetarians. *European Journal of Clinical Nutrition* 57, no. 2 (2003): 299–304.

Kynast-Gales, S. A., and L. K. Massey. Effect of caffeine on circadian excretion of urinary calcium and magnesium. *Journal of the American College of Nutrition* 13, no. 5 (1994): 467–72.

———. Effects of dietary calcium from dairy products on ambulatory blood pressure in hypertensive men. *Journal of the American Dietetic Association* 92, no. 12 (1992): 1497–1501.

Lin, P., M. Aickin, C. Champagne, S. Craddick, F. M. Sacks, P. McCarron,

M. M. Most-Windhauser, F. Rukenbrod, and L. Haworth. Food group sources of nutrients in the dietary patterns of the DASH-Sodium trial. *Journal of the American Dietetic Association* 103, no. 4 (2003): 488–96.

Massey, L. K. Dairy food consumption, blood pressure, and stroke. *The Journal of Nutrition* 131, no. 7 (2001): 1875–78.

McCarron, P. B. Dietary approaches to stop hypertension. *American Dietetic Association Sports, Cardiovascular and Wellness Nutritionists Dietetic Practice Group Pulse Newsletter* 21, no. 3 (2002): 1–3.

Mu, J. J., Z. Q. Liu, J. Yang, Y. M. Liang, D. J. Zhy, Y. X. Wang, B. L. Gao, X. L. Zhang, H. C. Ji, and X. L. Xu. Long-term observation in effects of potassium and calcium supplementation on arterial blood pressure and sodium metabolism in adolescents with higher blood pressure. *Chinese Journal of Preventative Medicine* 37, no. 2 (2003): 90–92.

Pamnani, M. B., H. J. Bryant, D. L. Clough, and J. F. Schooley. Increased dietary potassium and magnesium attenuate experimental volume dependent hypertension possible through endogenous sodium-potassium pump inhibitor. *Clinical and Experimental Hypertension* 25, no. 2 (2003): 103–15.

Phillips, K. M., K. K. Stewart, N. M. Karanja, M. M. Windhauser, C. M. Champagne, J. F. Swain, P. H. Lin, and M. A. Evans. Validation of diet composition for the Dietary Approaches to Stop Hypertension trial. DASH Collaborative Research Group. *Journal of the American Dietetic Association* 99, suppl. no 8 (1999): S60–S68.

Premier Collaborative Research Group. Effects of comprehensive lifestyle modification on blood pressure control. *Journal of the American Medical Association* 289 (2003): 2083–93.

Reynolds, K., L. B. Lewis, J. D. L. Nolen, G. L. Kinney, B. Sathya, and J. He. Alcohol consumption and risk of stroke. *Journal of the American Medical Association* 289 (2003): 579–88.

Sacco, R. L., M. Elkind, B. Boden-Albala, I. F. Lin, D. E. Kargman, W. A. Hauser, S. Shea, and M. C. Paik. The protective effect of moderate alcohol consumption on ischemic stroke. *Journal of the American Medical Association* 281, no. 1 (1999): 53–60.

Sacks, F. M., L. P. Svetkey, W. M. Vollmer, L. J. Appel, G. A. Bray, D. Harsha, E. Obarzanek, P. R. Conlin, E. R. Miller III, D. G. Simons-Morton, N. Karanja, P. H. Lin, D.A.-S.C.R. Group. Effects on blood pressure of reduced dietary sodium and the Dietary Approaches to Stop Hypertension (DASH) diet. DASH-Sodium Collaborative Research Group. *New England Journal of Medicine* 344, no. 3 (2001): 3–10.

Spence, J. D. Nutritional and metabolic aspects of stroke prevention. *Advances in Neurology* 92 (2003): 173–78.

Svetkey, L. P., F. M. Sacks, E. Obarzanek, W. M. Vollmer, L. J. Appel, P. H. Lin, N. M. Karanja, D. W. Harsha, G. A. Bray, M. Aickin, M. A. Proschan,

M. M. Windhauser, J. F. Swain, P. B. McCarron, D. G. Rhodes, and R. L. Laws. The DASH Diet, sodium intake and blood pressure trial (DASH-sodium): Rationale and design. DASH-Sodium Collaborative Research Group. *Journal of the American Dietetic Association* 99, suppl no. 8 (1999): S96–S104.

Touyz, R. M. Role of magnesium in the pathogenesis of hypertension. *Molecular Aspects of Medicine* 24, nos. 1–3 (2003): 107–36.

U.S. Department of Health and Human Services. National Institutes of Health. National Heart, Lung, and Blood Institute. *Facts About the DASH Eating Plan.* Washington, D.C.: U.S. Department of Health and Human Services, 2003, 11–23.

———. National Institutes of Health. *The Seventh Report of the Joint National Committee on Prevention, Detection, Evaluation, and Treatment of High Blood Pressure.* Washington, D.C.: U.S. Department of Health and Human Services, 2003, 1–34.

Vlachopoulos, C., K. Hirata, C. Stefanadis, P. Toutouzas, and M. F. O'Rourke. Caffeine increases aortic stiffness in hypertensive patients. *American Journal of Hypertension* 16, no. 1 (2003): 63–66.

Wise, K. J., E. A. Bergman, D. J. Sherrard, and L. K. Massey. Interactions between dietary calcium and caffeine on calcium metabolism in hypertensive humans. *American Journal of Hypertension* 9, no. 3 (1996): 223–29.

Writing Group of the PREMIER Collaborative Research Group. Effects of comprehensive lifestyle modification on blood pressure control. *Journal of the American Medical Association* 289, no. 16 (2003): 2083–93.

Yamori, Y., L. Liu, L. Mu, H. Zhao, Y. Pen, Z. Hu, S. Kuga, H. Negishi, and K. Ikeda. Diet-related factors, educational levels, and blood pressure in a Chinese population sample: Findings from the Japan-China Cooperative Research Project. *Hypertension Research* 25, no. 4 (2002): 559–64.

CHAPTER 6: PHENOTYPE C

Adank, C., T. J. Green, C. M. Skeaff, and B. Briars. Weekly high-dose folic acid supplementation is effective in lowering serum homocysteine concentrations in women. *Annals of Nutrition & Metabolism* 47 (2003): 55–59.

American Dietetic Association. Health implications of dietary fiber. *Journal of the American Dietetic Association* 102, no. 7 (2002): 993–1000.

American Heart Association. 2001 Heart & Stroke Statistical Update. Dallas: American Heart Association, 2001.

Anderson, J. W., L. D. Allgood, J. Turner, P. R. Oeltgen, and B. P. Daggy. Effects of psyllium on glucose and serum lipid responses in men with type

2 diabetes and hypercholesterolemia. *American Journal of Clinical Nutrition* 70, no. 4 (1999): 466–73.

Antonio, J., C. M. Colker, G. C. Torina, et al. Effects of a standardized guggulsterone phosphate supplement on body composition in overweight adults: a pilot study. *Current Therapeutic Research* 60 (1999): 220–27.

Balentine, D. A., M. C. Albano, and G. Muraleedharan. Role of medicinal plants, herbs, and spices in protecting human health. *Nutrition Reviews* 557 (1999): S41–S45.

Bazzano, L. A., J. He, L. G. Ogden, C. M. Loria, S. Vupputuri, L. Myers, and P. K. Whelton. Fruit and vegetable intake and risk of cardiovascular disease in U.S. adults: The first National Health and Nutrition Examination Survey Epidemiologic Follow-up Study. *American Journal of Clinical Nutrition* 76 (2002): 93–99.

Blair, S. N., D. M. Capuzzi, S. O. Gottlieb, T. Nguyen, J. M. Morgan, and N. B. Cater. Incremental reduction of serum total cholesterol and low-density lipoprotein cholesterol with the addition of plant stanol ester-containint spread to statin therapy. *The American Journal of Cardiology* 86 (2000): 46–52.

Bredie, S. J. H., C. J. J. Tack, P. Smits, and A. F. H. Stalenhoef. Nonobese patients with familial combined hyperlipidemia are insulin resistant compared with their nonaffected relatives. *Arteriosclerosis, Thrombosis, and Vascular Biology* 17 (1997): 1465–71.

Brown, L., B. Rosner, W. W. Willett, and F. M. Sacks. Cholesterol-lowering effects of dietary fiber: a meta-analysis. *American Journal of Clinical Nutrition* 69, no. 1 (1999): 30–42.

Bruunsgaard, H., H. E. Poulsen, B. K. Pedersen, K. Nyyssönen, J. Kaikkonen, and J. T. Salonen. Long-term combined supplementations with alpha-tocopherol and vitamin C have no detectable anti-inflammatory effects in healthy men. *The Journal of Nutrition* 133, no. 4 (2003): 1170–73.

Caron, M. F., and C. M. White. Evaluation of the antihyperlipidemic properties of dietary supplements. *Pharmacotherapy* 21, no. 4 (2001): 481–87.

Castano, G., R. Mas, L. Fernandez, R. Gamez, and J. Illnait. Effects of policosanol and lovastatin in patients with intermittent claudication: A double-blind comparative pilot study. *Angiology* 54, no. 1 (2003): 25–38.

Cater, N. B., and S. M. Grundy. Lowering serum cholesterol with plant sterols and stanols. *Postgraduate Medicine*, 1998, 6–14.

Church, T. S., C. E. Barlow, C. P. Earnest, J. B. Kampert, E. L. Priest, and S. N. Blair. Associations between cardiorespiratory fitness and C-reactive protein in men. *Arteriosclerosis, Thrombosis, and Vascular Biology* 22, no. 11 (2002): 869–76.

Cui, J., L. Huang, A. Zhao, J. L. Lew, J. Yu, S. Sahoo, P. T. Meinke, I. Royo, F. Pelaez, and S. D. Wright. Guggulsterone is a farnesoid X receptor antagonist in coactivator association assays but acts to enhance transcription of bile salt export pump. *Journal of Biological Chemistry* 278, no. 12 (2003): 10,214–20.

Danesh, J., R. Collins, P. Appleby, and R. Peto. Association of fibrinogen, C-reactive protein, albumin, or leukocyte count with coronary heart disease: Meta-analyses of prospective studies. *Journal of the American Medical Association* 279 (1998): 1477–82.

Davi, G., M. T. Guagnano, G. Ciabattoni, S. Basili, A. Falco, M. Marinopiccoli, M. Nutini, S. Sensi, and C. Patrono. Platelet activation in obese women. *Journal of the American Medical Association* 288, no. 16 (2002): 2008–14.

Davidson, M. H., and C. T. Geohas. Efficacy of over-the-counter nutritional supplements. *Current Atherosclerosis Report* 5, no. 1 (2003): 15–21.

DeBusk, R. F., U. Sendestrand, M. Sheehan, and W. L. Haskell. Training effects of long versus short bouts of exercise in healthy subjects. *The American Journal of Cardiology* 65, no. 15 (1990): 1010–13.

Diebolt, M., B. Bucher, and R. Andriantsitohaina. Wine polyphenols decrease blood pressure, improve NO vasodialation, and induce gene expression. *Hypertension* 38 (2001): 159–65.

Efendy, J. L., D. L. Simmons, G. R. Campbell, et al. The effect of the aged garlic extract, "Kyolic," on the development of experimental atherosclerosis. *Atherosclerosis* 132 (1997): 37–42.

Esposito, K., A. Pontillo, C. Di Palo, G. Giugliano, M. Masella, R. Marfella, and D. Giugliano. Effect of weight loss and lifestyle changes on vascular inflammatory markers in obese women. *Journal of the American Medical Association* 289, no. 14 (2003): 1799–1804.

Extra co-enzyme Q10 for statin-users? *Treatment Update* 13, no. 2 (2001): 4–7.

Folts, J. D., B. Begolli, et al. Inhibition of platelet activity with red wine and grape products. *Biofactors* 6, no. 4 (1997): 411–14.

Freedman, J. E., P. L. Crawford, L. Liqing, et al. Select flavonoids and whole juice from purple grapes inhibit platelet function. *Circulation* 103 (2001): 2792–98.

Gardner, C. D., L. M. Chatterjee, and J. J. Carlson. The effect of a garlic preparation on plasma lipid levels in moderately hypercholesterolemic adults. *Atherosclerosis* 154 (2001): 213–20.

Gouni-Berthold, I., H. K. Berthold. Policosanol: clinical pharmacology and therapeutic significance of a new lipid-lowering agent. *American Heart Journal* 143, no. 2 (2002): 356–65.

Grundy, S. M., R. Pasternak, P. Greenland, S. Smith Jr., and V. Fuster.

AHA/ACC scientific statement: Assessment of cardiovascular risk by use of multiple risk factor assessment equations: a statement for healthcare professionals from the American Heart Association and the American College of Cardiology. *Journal of the American College of Cardiology* 34 (1999): 1348–59.

Hannum, S. M., H. H. Schmitz, and C. L. Keen. Chocolate: A heart-healthy food? Show me the science! *Nutrition Today* 37, no. 3 (2002): 103–9.

Harris, W. S. N-3 fatty acids and serum lipoproteins: Human studies. *American Journal of Clinical Nutrition* 65, suppl. no 5 (1997): S1645–S1654.

Heales, S., and I. P. Hargreaves. Statins and myopathy. *The Lancet* 359, no. 9307 (2002): 711.

Hirschhorn, J. N., K. Lohmueller, E. Byrne, and K. Hirschhorn. A comprehensive review of genetic association studies. *Genetic Medicine* 4, no. 2 (2002): 45–61.

Holt, R. R., S. A. Lazarus, M. C. Sullards, Q. Y. Zhu, D. D. Schramm, J. F. Hammerstone, C. G. Fraga, H. H. Schmitz, and C. L. Keen. Procyanidin dimmer B2 [epicatechin- (4beta-8) -epicatechin] in human plasma after the consumption of a flavonol-rich cocoa. *American Journal of Clinical Nutrition* 76, no. 4 (2002): 798–804.

Howard, B. V., and D. Kritchevsky. Phytochemicals and cardiovascular disease. *Circulation* 95 (1997): 2591–93.

Ichihara, K., and K. Satoh. Disparity between angiographic regression and clinical event rates with hydrophobic statins. *The Lancet* 359, no. 9324 (2002): 2195.

Janikula, M. Policosanol: A new treatment for cardiovascular disease? *Alternative Medicine Review* 7, no. 3 (2002): 203–17.

Jenkins, D. J., C. W. Kendall, V. Vuksan, et al. Soluble fiber intake at a dose approved by the U.S. Food and Drug Administration for a claim of health benefits: Serum lipid risk factors for cardiovascular disease assessed in a randomized controlled crossover trial. *American Journal of Clinical Nutrition* 75, no. 5 (2002): 834–39.

Jiang, Q., and B. N. Ames. Gamma-tocopherol, but not alpha-tocopherol, decreases proinflammatory eicosanoids and inflammation damage in rats. *The FASEB Journal* 17, no. 8 (2003): 816–22.

Jiang, Q., S. Christen, M. K. Shigenaga, and B. N. Ames. Gamma-tocopherol, the major form of vitamin E in the U.S. diet, deserves more attention. *American Journal of Clinical Nutrition* 74 (2001): 714–22.

Jimenez-Sanchez, G., B. Childs, and D. Valle. Human disease genes. *Nature* 409 (2001): 853–55.

Kannar, D., N. Wattanapenpaiboon, G. S. Savige, et al. Hypocholesterolemic effect of an enteric coated garlic supplement. *Journal of the American College of Nutrition* 20 (2001): 225–31.

Keen, C. L. Chocolate: Food as medicine/medicine as food. *Journal of the American College of Nutrition* 20, suppl. no. 5 (2001): 436S–439S.

Krauss, R. M. Dietary and genetic effects on low-density lipoprotein heterogeneity. *Annual Review of Nutrition* 21 (2001): 283–95.

Kris-Etherton, P. M. AHA Science Advisory. Monounsaturated fatty acids and risk of cardiovascular disease. *Circulation* 100 (1999): 1253–58.

Kris-Etherton, P. M., and C. L. Keen. Evidence that the antioxidant flavonoids in tea and cocoa are beneficial for cardiovascular health. *Current Opinion in Lipidology* 13, no. 1 (2002): 41–49.

Kris-Etherton, P. M., W. S. Harris, and L. J. Appel for the Nutrition Committee. American Heart Association Scientific Statement. Fish consumption, fish oil, omega-3 fatty acids, and cardiovascular disease. *Circulation* 106 (2002): 2747–57.

Kris-Etherton, P. M., T. A. Pearson, Y. Wan, et al. High-monounsaturated fatty acid diets lower both plasma cholesterol and triacylglycerol concentrations. *American Journal of Clinical Nutrition* 70 (1999): 1009–15.

Manson, J. E., G. A. Colditz, M. J. Stampfer, et al. A prospective study of obesity and the risk of coronary heart disease in women. *New England Journal of Medicine* 332 (1990): 882–89.

Masson, L. F., G. McNeill, A. Avenell. Genetic variation and the lipid response to dietary intervention: A systematic review. *American Journal of Clinical Nutrition* 77, no. 5 (2003): 1098–1111.

Mensink, R. P., and J. Plat. Efficacy of dietary plant stanols. *Postgraduate Medicine,* 1998, 27–31.

Miettinen, T. A., P. Puska, H. Gylling, H. Vanhanen, E. Vartiainen. Reduction of serum cholesterol with sitostanol-ester margarine in a mildly hypercholesterolemic population. *New England Journal of Medicine* 333 (1995): 1308–12.

National Cholesterol Education Program (NCEP). Executive summary of the third report of the expert panel on detection, evaluation, and treatment of high blood cholesterol in adults. *Journal of the American Medical Association* 285 (2001): 2486–97.

National Institutes of Health, National Heart, Lung, and Blood Institute. *Third Report of the National Cholesterol Education Program (NCEP) Expert Panel on Detection, Evaluation, and Treatment of High Blood Cholesterol in Adults (Adult Treatment Panel III).* NIH Publication, 2001.

Nilsen, D. W., G. Albrektsen, K. Landmark, et al. Effects of high-dose concentrate of n-3 fatty acids or corn oil introduced early after an acute myocardial infarction on serum triacylglycerol and HDL cholesterol. *American Journal of Clinical Nutrition* 74 (2001): 50–56.

O'Brien, T., and T. T. Nguyen. Lipids and lipoproteins in women. *Mayo Clinic Proceedings* 72 (1997): 235–44.

O'Byrne, D. J., S. Devaraj, S. M. Grundy, and I. Jialal. Comparison of the antioxidant effects of Concord grape juice flavonoids alpha-tocopherol on markers of oxidative stress in healthy adults. *American Journal of Clinical Nutrition* 76, no. 6 (2002): 1367–74.

Ordovas, J. M., D. Corella, L. A. Cuppies, S. Demissie, A. Kelleher, O. Coltell, P. W. Wilson, E. J. Schaefer, and K. Tucker. Polyunsaturated fatty acids modulate the effects of the APOA1 G-A polymorphism on HDL-cholesterol concentrations in a sex-specific manner: The Framingham Study. *American Journal of Clinical Nutrition* 75, no. 1 (2002): 38–46.

Pearce, K. A., M. G. Boosalis, and B. Yeager. Update on vitamin supplements for the prevention of coronary disease and stroke. *American Family Physician* 62, no. 6 (2000): 1359–67.

Pearson, T. A., S. N. Blair, S. R. Daniels, R. H. Eckel, J. M. Fair, S. P. Fortmann, B. A. Franklin, L. B. Goldstein, P. Greenland, S. M. Grundy, Y. Hong, N. H. Miller, R. M. Lauer, I. S. Ockene, R. L. Sacco, J. F. Sallis Jr., S. C. Smith Jr., N. J. Stone, and K. A. Taubert. AHA guidelines for primary prevention of cardiovascular disease and stroke: 2002 Update: Consensus panel guide to comprehensive risk reduction for adult patients without coronary or other atherosclerotic vascular diseases. American Heart Association Science Advisory and Coordinating Committee. *Circulation* 106 (2002): 388–91.

Rein, D., T. G. Paglieroni, T. Wun, D. A. Pearson, H. H. Schmitz, R. Gosselin, and C. L. Keen. Cocoa inhibits platelet activation and function. *American Journal of Clinical Nutrition* 72, no. 1 (2000): 30–35.

Ridker, P. M., N. Rifai, L. Rose, J. E. Buring, and N. R. Cook. Comparison of C-reactive protein and low-density lipoprotein cholesterol levels in the prediction of first cardiovascular events. *New England Journal of Medicine* 347, no. 20 (2002): 1557–65.

Safeer, R. S., and P. S. Ugalat. Cholesterol treatment guidelines update. *American Family Physician* 65, no. 5 (2002): 871–80.

Seeram, N. P., R. A. Momin, M. G. Nair, and L. D. Bourquin. Cyclooxygenase inhibitory and antioxidant cyanidin glycosides in cherries and berries. *Phytomedicine* 8, no. 5 (2001): 362–69.

Singh, R. B., M. A. Niaz, and S. Ghosh. Hypolipidemic and antioxidant effects of *Commiphora mukul* as an adjunct to dietary therapy in patients with hypercholesterolemia. *Cardiovascular Drugs and Therapy* 8 (1994): 659–64.

Slap, J. K. Effects of psyllium on serum lipids. *American Journal of Clinical Nutrition* 68, no. 4 (1998): 923–24.

Steinberg, F. M., M. M. Bearden, and C. L. Keen. Cocoa and chocolate flavonoids: Implications for cardiovascular health. *Journal of the American Dietetic Association* 103, no. 2 (2003): 215–23.

Stevinson, C., M. H. Pittler, and E. Ernst. Garlic for treating hypercholesterolemia. A meta-analysis of randomized clinical trials. *Annals of Internal Medicine* 133 (2000): 420–29.

Stoll, A. L., W. E. Severus, M. P. Freeman, et al. Omega-3 fatty acids in bipolar disorder: A preliminary double-blind, placebo-controlled trial. *Archives of General Psychiatry* 56 (1999): 407–12.

Urizar, N. L., A. B. Liverman, D. T. Dodds, F. V. Silva, P. Ordentlich, Y. Yan, F. J. Gonzalez, R. A. Heyman, D. J. Mangelsdorf, and D. D. Moore. A natural product that lowers cholesterol as an antagonist ligand for FXR. *Science* 296, no. 5573 (2002): 1703–6.

Urizar, N. L., and D. D. Moore. Gugulipid: A natural cholesterol-lowering agent. *Annual Review of Nutrition* 23 (2003): 303–13.

Van Dam, M., A. F. Stalenhoef, J. Wittekoek, et al. Efficacy of concentrated n-3 fatty acids in hypertriglyceridaemia: A comparison with gemfibrozil. *Clinical Drug Investigation* 21 (2001): 175–81.

Van Horn, L., and N. Ernst. A summary of the science supporting the new national cholesterol education program dietary recommendations: What dietitians should know. *Journal of the American Dietetic Association* 101, no. 10 (2001): 1148–54.

Vanschoonbeek, K., M. P. M. de Maat, and J. W. M. Heemskerk. Fish oil consumption and reduction of arterial disease. *The Journal of Nutrition* 133 (2003): 657–60.

Visser, M., L. M. Bouter, G. M. McQuillan, M. H. Wener, and T. B. Harris. Elevated C-reactive protein levels in overweight and obese adults. *Journal of the American Medical Association* 282, no. 22 (1999): 2131–35.

Von Bergmann, K., and D. Lutjohann. Review of the absorption and safety of plant sterols. *Postgraduate Medicine,* 1998, 54–59.

Von Schacky, C., P. Angerer, W. Kothny, et al. The effect of dietary omega-3 fatty acids on coronary atherosclerosis. A randomized, double-blind, placebo-controlled trial. *Annals of Internal Medicine* 130 (1999): 554–62.

Webb, Denise, for Environmental Nutrition. From starring role to bit part: Has the curtain come down on vitamin E? *The Newsletter of Food, Nutrition & Health* 25, no. 5 (2002).

Wu, J. M., Z. R. Wang, T. C. Hsieh, J. L. Bruder, J. G. Zou, and Y. Z. Huang. Mechanisms of cardioprotection by resveratrol, a phenolic antioxidant present in red wine. *International Journal of Molecular Medicine* 8 (2002): 3–17.

Yang, C. S., and J. M. Landau. Effects of tea consumption on nutrition and health. *The Journal of Nutrition* 132 (2002): 2409–12.

CHAPTER 7: PHENOTYPE D

Althuis, M. D., N. E. Jordan, E. A. Ludington, and J. T. Wittes. Glucose and insulin responses to dietary chromium supplements: A meta-analysis. *American Journal of Clinical Nutrition* 76 (2002): 148–55.

American Diabetes Association. Evidence-based nutrition principles and recommendations for the treatment and prevention of diabetes and related complications. *Diabetes Care* 26, suppl. no. 1 (2003): S51–S61.

———. Diabetes mellitus and exercise. Position statement. *Diabetes Care* 25, suppl. no. 1 (2002): S64–S68.

———. Nutrition recommendations and principles for people with diabetes mellitus. Position statement. *Diabetes Care* 23, suppl. no. 1 (2000): 543–46.

Anderson, J. W., L. D. Allgood, J. Turner, P. R. Oeltgen, and B. P. Daggy. Effects of psyllium on glucose and serum lipid responses in men with type 2 diabetes and hypercholesterolemia. *American Journal of Clinical Nutrition* 70, no. 4 (1999): 466.

Antioxidants make sense as adjunct therapy for type 2 diabetes. *Diabetes Week,* March 28, 2003, 4.

Baba, N. H., S. Sawaya, H. Torbay, Z. Habbal, S. Azar, and S. A. Hashim. High protein vs high carbohydrate hypoenergetic diet for the treatment of obese hyperinsulinemic subjects. *International Journal of Obesity and Related Metabolic Disorders* 23 (1999): 1202–06.

Barringer, T. A., J. K. Kirk, A. C. Santaniello, K. L. Foley, and R. Michielutte. Effect of a multivitamin and mineral supplement on infection and quality of life. A randomized, double-blind, placebo-controlled trial. *Annals of Internal Medicine* 138, no. 5 (2003): 365–71.

Basch, E., C. Ulbricht, G. Kuo, P. Szapary, and M. Smith. Therapeutic applications of Fenugreek. *Alternative Medicine Review* 8, no. 1 (2003): 20–27.

Boeing, H., U. M. Weisgerber, A. Jeckel, H. J. Rose, and A. Kroke. Association between glycated hemoglobin and diet and other lifestyle factors in a nondiabetic population: Cross-sectional evaluation of data from the Potsdam cohort of the European Prospective Investigation into Cancer and Nutrition Study. *American Journal of Clinical Nutrition* 71, no. 5 (2000): 1115–22.

Brand-Miller, J. C., S. H. Holt, D. B. Pawlak, and J. McMillan. Glycemic index and obesity. *American Journal of Clinical Nutrition* 76, no. 1 (2002): 281S–285S.

Chandalia, M., A. Garg, D. Lutjohann, K. von Bergmann, S. M. Grundy, and L. J. Brinkley. Beneficial effects of high dietary fiber intake in patients with type 2 diabetes mellitus. *New England Journal of Medicine* 342 (2000): 1392–98.

DiSilvestro, R. A. Zinc in relation to diabetes and oxidative disease. *The Journal of Nutrition* 130, no. 5 (2000): 1509S–1511S.

Foster-Powell, K., S. H. Holt, and J. C. Brand-Miller. International table of glycemic index and glycemic load values: 2002. *American Journal of Clinical Nutrition* 76, no. 1 (2002): 5–56.

Franz, M. J., J. P. Bantle, C. A. Beebe, J. D. Brunzell, J. L. Chiasson, A. Garg, L. A. Holzmeister, B. Hoogwerf, E. Mayer-Davis, A. D. Mooradian, J. Q. Purnell, and M. Wheeler. Evidence-based nutrition principles and recommendations for the treatment and prevention of diabetes and related complications. Technical review. *Diabetes Care* 25 (2002): 148–98.

Garg, A. High-monounsaturated-fat diets for patients with diabetes mellitus: A meta-analysis. *American Journal of Clinical Nutrition* 67, suppl. no. 3 (1998): 577S–582S.

Guerrero-Romero, F., and M. Rodriguez-Moran. Low serum magnesium levels and metabolic syndrome. *Acta Diabetologica* 39, no. 4 (2002): 209–13.

Hu, F. B., J. E. Manson, M. J. Stampfer, G. Colditz, S. Liu, C. G. Solomon, and W. C. Willett. Diet, lifestyle, and the risk of type 2 diabetes mellitus in women. *New England Journal of Medicine* 345, no. 11 (2001): 790–97.

Il'Yasova, D., L. Wagenknecht, and J. Morrow. Free radicals and incident type 2 diabetes: A case-control study nested in the Insulin Resistance Atherosclerosis Study (IRAS). *Diabetes* 52, no. 6 (2003): A222.

Jayagopal, V., P. Albertazzi, E. S. Kilpatrick, E. M. Howarth, P. E. Jennings, D. A. Hepburn, and S. L. Atkin. Beneficial effects of soy phytoestrogen intake in postmenopausal women with type 2 diabetes. *Diabetes Care* 25, no. 10 (2002): 1709–14.

Jenkins, D. J., C. W. Kendall, L. S. Augustin, S. Franceschi, M. Hamidi, A. Marchie, A. L. Jenkins, and M. Axelsen. Glycemic index: Overview of implications in health and disease. *American Journal of Clinical Nutrition* 76, no. 1 (2002): 266S–273S.

Kahn, C. R. Banting lecture: Insulin action, diabetogenes, and the cause of type 2 diabetes. *Diabetes* 43 (1994): 1066–84.

Kantor, L. S., J. N. Variyam, J. E. Allshouse, J. J. Putnam, and B. H. Lin. Choose a variety of grains daily, especially whole grains: A challenge for consumers. *The Journal of Nutrition* 131 (2001): S473–S486.

Kim, M., J. Park, H. Park, J. Youn, M. Shin, C. Namkoong, and K. I. Lee. Chronic administration of a-lipoic acid prevents diabetes mellitus in obese OLETF rats. *Diabetes* 52, no. 6 (2003): A123.

Latner, J. D., and M. Schwartz. The effects of a high-carbohydrate, high-protein or balanced lunch upon later food intake and hunger ratings. *Appetite* 33 (1999): 119–28.

Leeds, A. R. Glycemic index and heart disease. *American Journal of Clinical Nutrition* 76, no. 1 (2002): 286S–289S.

Lipkin, E. New strategies for the treatment of type 2 diabetes. *Journal of the American Dietetic Association* 99, no. 3 (1999): 329–33.

Liu, S., J. E. Manson, M. J. Stampfer, F. B. Hu, E. Giovannucci, G. A. Colditz, C. H. Hennekens, and W. C. Willett. A prospective study of whole-grain intake and risk of type 2 diabetes mellitus in U.S. women. *American Journal of Public Health* 90 (2000): 1409–15.

Lonn, E., S. Yusuf, B. Hoogwerf, J. Pogue, Q. Yi, B. Zinman, J. Bosch, G. Dagenais, J. F. E. Mann, and H. C. Gerstein. Effects of vitamin E on cardiovascular and microvascular outcomes in high-risk patients with diabetes. *Diabetes Care* 25 (2002): 1919–27.

Meigs, J. B. Invited commentary: Insulin resistance syndrome? Syndrome X? Multiple metabolic syndrome? A syndrome at all? Factor analysis reveals patterns in the fabric of correlated metabolic risk factors. *American Journal of Epidemiology* 152 (2000): 908–11.

Park, S. and S. B. Choi. Effects of [alpha]-tocopherol supplementation and continuous subcutaneous insulin infusion on oxidative stress in Korean patients with type 2 diabetes. *American Journal of Clinical Nutrition* 75, no. 4 (2002): 728–33.

Parker, B., M. Noakes, N. Luscombe, and P. Clifton. Effect of a high-protein, high-monounsaturated fat weight loss diet on glycemic control and lipid levels in type 2 diabetes. *Diabetes Care* 25, no. 3 (2002): 425–30.

Pi-Sunyer, F. X. Glycemic index and disease. *American Journal of Clinical Nutrition* 76, no. 1 (2002): 290S–298S.

Robertson, R. P., J. Harmon, P. O. Tran, Y. Tanaka, and H. Takahashi. Glucose toxicity in [beta]-cells: Type 2 diabetes, good radicals gone bad, and the glutathione connection. *Diabetes* 52, no. 3 (2003): 581–87.

Rodriguez-Moran, M. and F. Guerrero-Romero. Oral magnesium supplementation improves insulin sensitivity and metabolic control in type 2 diabetic subjects. *Diabetes Care* 26 (2003): 1147–52.

Roussel, A., A. Kerkeni, N. Zouari, S. Mahjoub, J. Matheau, and R. A. Anderson. Antioxidant effects of zinc supplementation in Tunisians with type 2 diabetes mellitus. *Journal of the American College of Nutrition* 22, no. 4 (2003): 316–21.

Sacks, F. M., L. P. Svetkey, W. M. Vollmer, L. J. Appel, G. A. Bray, D. Harsha, E. Obarzanek, P. R. Conlin, E. R. Miller, D. G. Simons-Morton, N. Karanja, and P. H. Lin, for the DASH-Sodium Collaborative Research Group. Effects on blood pressure of reduced dietary sodium and the dietary approaches to stop hypertension (DASH) diet. *New England Journal of Medicine* 344 (2001): 3–10.

Sarubin, A. You need more vitamin C: Current RDA offers less than maximum protection from cancer, diabetes, and more. *Prevention* 54, no. 12 (2002): 71–72.

Schefrin, R. Good carbs, bad carbs. *Today's Dietitian* 5, no. 4 (2003): 36–39.

Sierra, M., J. J. Garcia, and N. Fernandez. Therapeutic effects of psyllium in type 2 diabetic patients. *Alternative Medicine Review* 7, no. 6 (2002): 541(1).

Skov, A. R., S. Toubro, B. Ronn, L. Holm, and A. Astrup. Randomized trial on protein vs carbohydrate in ad libitum fat reduced diet for the treatment of obesity. *International Journal of Obesity and Related Metabolic Disorders* 23 (1999): 528–36.

Tuomilehto, J., J. Lindstrom, J. G. Eriksson, T. T. Valle, H. Hamalainen, P. Ilanne-Parikka, S. Keinanen-Kiukaanniemi, M. Laakso, A. Louheranta, M. Rastas, V. Salminen, M. Uusitupa, S. Aunola, Z. Cepaitis, V. Moltchanov, M. Hakumaki, M. Mannelin, V. Martikkala, and J. Sundvall. Prevention of type 2 diabetes mellitus by changes in lifestyle amount subjects with impaired glucose tolerance. *New England Journal of Medicine* 344 (2001): 1343–50.

Vitamins C and E may enhance effectiveness of insulin for diabetes. *Diabetes Week,* January 17, 2003, 18.

Willett, W., J. Manson, and S. Liu. Glycemic index, glycemic load, and risk of type 2 diabetes. *American Journal of Clinical Nutrition* 76, no. 1 (2002): 274S–280S.

Wolfe, B. M., and P. M. Giovanetti. Short-term effects of substituting protein for carbohydrate in the diets of moderately hypercholesterolemic human subjects. *Metabolism* 40 (1991): 338–43.

Yeh, G. Y., D. M. Eisenberg, T. J. Kaptchuk, and R. S. Phillips. Systematic review of herbs and dietary supplements for glycemic control in diabetes. *Diabetes Care* 26 (2003): 1277–94.

Ylonen, K., G. Alfthan, L. Groop, C. Saloranta, A. Aro, and S. M. Virtanen. Dietary intakes and plasma concentrations of carotenoids and tocopherols in relation to glucose metabolism in subjects at high risk of type 2 diabetes: The Botnia Dietary Study. *American Journal of Clinical Nutrition* 77, no. 6 (2003): 1434–41.

CHAPTER 8: PHENOTYPE E

Barr, S. I. Increased dairy product or calcium intake: Is body weight or composition affected in humans? *The Journal of Nutrition* 133, no. 1 (2003): 245S–254S.

Bruinsma, K. A., D. L. Taren. Dieting, essential fatty acid intake and depression. *Nutrition Reviews* 58 (2000): 98–108.

Byerly, W. F., et al. 5-hydroxytryptophan: A review of its antidepressant efficacy and adverse effects. *Journal of Clinical Psychopharmacology* 7 (1987): 127–137.

Clairmont, M. A. Fitness for all sizes. *Today's Dietitian* 5, no. 4 (2003): 33–35.

Cohen, J. H., A. R. Kristal, D. Neumark-Sztainer, C. L. Rock, M. L. Neuhouser. Psychological distress is associated with unhealthful dietary practices. *Journal of the American Dietetic Association* 102, no. 5 (2002): 699–703.

Foster, S., V. E. Tyler. *Tyler's Honest Herbal,* 4th edition. Binghamton: The Haworth Herbal Press, 1999.

Keller, J. R. Omega-3 fatty acids may be effective in the treatment of depression. *Topics in Clinical Nutrition* 17, no. 5 (2002): 21–27.

Laitinen, J., E. Ek, U. Sovio. Stress-related eating and drinking behavior and body mass index and predictors of this behavior. *Preventitive Medicine* 34, no. 1 (2002): 29–39.

Peet, M., D. E. Horrobin. A dose ranging study of the effects of ethyleicosapentaenoate in patients with ongoing depression despite apparently adequate treatment with standard drugs. *Archives of General Psychiatry* 59 (2002): 913–19.

Pinaquy, S., H. Chabrol, C. Simon, J. P. Louvet, and P. Barbe. Emotional eating, alexithymia, and binge-eating disorder in obese women. *Obesity Research* 11, no. 2 (2003): 195–201.

Schulz, V., R. Hansel, V. E. Tyler. *Rational Phytotherapy: A Physician's Guide to Herbal Medicine,* 3rd edition. Berlin: Springer-Veriag, 1998.

Soliah, L. A. The psychological appeal of fad diets. *Today's Dietitian* 5, no. 4 (2003): 22–24.

Tanskanen, A., J. R. Mibbelin, J. Hintikka, K. Haatainen, K. Honkalampi, H. Vinnamaki. Fish consumption, depression and suicidality in a general population. *Archives of General Psychiatry* 58 (2001): 512–513.

Teegarden, D. Calcium intake and reduction in weight or fat mass. *The Journal of Nutrition* 133, no. 1 (2003): 239S–253S.

Zemel, M. B., et al. Dietary calcium and dairy products accelerate weight and fat loss during energy restriction in obese adults. *American Journal of Clinical Nutrition* 75, no. 2 (2002): 342S.

Zemel, M. B. The mechanisms of dairy modulation of adiposity. *The Journal of Nutrition* 133, no. 1 (2003): 252S–255S.

CHAPTER 9: PHENOTYPE H

Burnette, M. M. et al. Smoking cessation, weight gain, and changes in cardiovascular risk factors during menopause: The healthy women study. *American Journal of Public Health* 88, no. 1 (1998): 93–96.

Chaverz, M. I., M. F. Spitzer. Herbals and other dietary supplements for premenstrual syndrome and menopause. *Psychiatric Annals* 32, no. 1 (2002): 61–74.

Carusi, D. Phytoestrogens as hormone replacement therapy: An evidence-based approach. *Primary Care Update for OB/GYNs* 7 no. 6 (2000): 253–259.

Condon, J. T. The premenstrual syndrome: A twin study. *British Journal of Psychiatry* 162 (1993): 481–486.

Despres, J. P., A. Tremblay, A. Nadeau, C. Bouchard. Physical training and changes in regional adipose tissue distribution. *Acta Medica Scandinavica Supplementum* 723 (1988): 205–207.

DeSouza, M. C., A. F. Walker, P. A. Robinson, et al. A synergistic effect of a daily supplement for one month of 200 mg magnesium plus 50 mg vitamin B-6 for the relief of anxiety-related premenstrual symptoms: A randomized double-blind, crossover study. *Journal of Women's Health and Gender Based Medicine* 9 (2000): 131–139.

Facchinetti, F., P. Borella, G. Sances, et al. Oral magnesium successfully relieves premenstrual mood changes. *Obstetrics & Gynecology* 78 (1991): 177–181.

Facchinetti, F., G. Sances, P. Borella, et al. Magnesium prophylaxis of menstrual migraine: Effects on intracellular magnesium. *Headache* 31 (1991): 298–301.

Feig, D. S., C. D. Naylor. Eating for two: Are guidelines for weight gain during pregnancy too liberal? *The Lancet* 351, no. 9108 (1998): 1054–55.

Ferrara, C. M., N. A. Lynch, B. J. Nicklas, A. S. Ryan, D. M. Berman. Differences in adipose tissue metabolism between postmenopausal and perimenopausal women. *Journal of Clinical Endocrinology & Metabolism* 87, no. 9 (2002): 4166–70.

Foster, S., V. E. Tyler. *Tyler's Honest Herbal,* 4th Edition. Binghamton: The Haworth Herbal Press, 1999.

Freeman, E. W., S. J. Sondheimer, K. Rickels. Effects of medical history factors on symptom severity in women meeting criteria for premenstrual syndrome. *Obstetrics & Gynecology* 72 (1988): 236–239.

Han, K. K., et al. Benefits of soy isoflavone therapeutic regimen on menopausal symptoms. *Obstetrics & Gynecology* 99, no. 3 (2002): 389–394.

Harris, H. E., G. T. H. Ellison, S. Clement. Relative importance of heritable characteristics and lifestyle in the development of maternal obesity. *Journal of Epidemiology and Community Health* 53, no. 2 (1999): 66.

Hinton, P. S., C. M. Olson, T. Peregrin. Postpartum exercise and food intake: The importance of behavior-specific self-efficacy. *Journal of the American Dietetic Association* 101, no. 12 (2001): 1430–1437.

Hirata, J. D., L. M. Swiersz, B. Zell, et al. Does dong quai have estrogenic effects in post-menopausal women? A double-blind placebo controlled trial. *Fertility and Sterility* 68 (1997): 981–986.

Jacobson, J. S., A. B. Troxel, J. Evans, et al. Randomized trial of black cohosh for the treatment of hot flashes among women with a history of breast cancer. *Journal of Clinical Oncology* 19 (2001): 2739–45.

Kendler, K. S., et al. Genetic and environmental factors in the etiology of menstrual, premenstrual, and neurotic symptoms: A population-based twin study. *Psychological Medicine* 22 (1992): 85–100.

Keppel, K., S. Taffel. Pregnancy-related weight gain and retention: Implications of the 1990 Institute of Medicine guidelines. *American Journal of Public Health* 83 (1993): 1100–1103.

Kramer, M. S., R. Kakuma. Optimal duration of exclusive breastfeeding. *Cochrane Database System Review,* no. 1 (2002): CD003517.

Kreydiyyeh, S. I., J. Usta. Diuretic effect and mechanism of action of parsley. *Journal of Ethnopharmacology* 79, no. 3 (2002): 353–7.

Kronenberg, F., A. Fugh-Berman. Complementary and alternative medicine for menopausal symptoms: A review of randomized, controlled trials. *Annals of Internal Medicine* 137 (2002): 805–813.

Leonetti, H. B., S. Longo, J. N. Anasti. Transdermal progesterone cream for vasomotor symptoms and post-menopausal bone loss. *American Journal of Obstetrics & Gynecology* 94 (1999): 225–228.

McCrory, M. Does dieting during lactation put infant growth at risk? *Nutrition Reviews.* 59, no. 1 (2001): 18–21.

Murphy, M. H., A. E. Hardeman. Training effects of short and long bouts of brisk walking in sedentary women. *Medicine and Science in Sports and Exercise* 30, no. 1 (1998): 152–7.

Nestel, P. J., S. Pomeroy, S. Kay, et al. Isoflavones from red clover improve systemic arterial compliance but not plasma lipids in menopausal women. *The Journal of Clinical Endocrinology & Metabolism* 84 (1999): 895–898.

Park, S. K., J. H. Park, Y. C. Kwon, H. S. Kim, M. S. Yoon, H. T. Park. The effect of combined aerobic and resistance exercise training on abdominal fat in obese middle-aged women. *Journal of Physiological Anthropology and Applied Human Science* 22, no. 3 (2003): 129–35.

Potter, S. M., J. A. Baum, H. Teng, et al. Soy protein and isoflavones: Their effects on blood lipids and bone density in postmenopausal women with low bone mass. *Calcified Tissue International* 54 (1994): 377–380.

Prabhakaran, B., E. A. Dowling, J. D. Branch, D. P. Swain, B. C. Leutholtz. Effects of 14 weeks of resistance training on lipid profile and body fat percentages in premenopausal women. *British Journal of Sports Medicine* 33, no. 3 (1999): 190–5.

Rooney, B. L., C. W. Schauberger. Excess pregnancy weight gain and long-term obesity: One decade later. *Obstetrics & Gynecology* 100, no. 2 (2002): 245–52.

Schellenberg, R. Treatment for the premenstrual syndrome with Agnus castus fruit extract: Prospective, randomized, placebo controlled study. *British Medical Journal* 322 (2001): 134–137.

Scholl, I. Q., M. L. Hediger, J. I. Schall, I. G. Ances, W. K. Smith. Gestational weight gain, pregnancy outcome, and postpartum weight retention. *Obstetrics & Gynecology* 86 (1995): 423–427.

Somvanshi, N. P. Preventing postpartum weight retention. *American Family Physician* 66, no. 3 (2002): 380–383.

Use of botanicals for management of menopausal symptoms. ACOG Practice Bulletin Number 28, June 2001. American College of Obstetricians and Gynecologists (409 12th Street SW, P.O. Box 96920, Washington, D.C. 20090–6920).

Weingarten, H. P. Food cravings in a college population. *Appetite* 17 (1991): 167–175.

Index

About the Authors

DR. SUSAN MITCHELL makes nutrition fun and healthy eating easy. A much sought after nutrition expert, she's been seen on *The Today Show, CNN, Weekend Today in New York,* and *The TV Food Network* and been quoted in magazines including *Reader's Digest, Time, Cooking Light, Redbook,* and *Fitness.*

A fellow of the American Dietetic Association, registered dietitian, and certified nutrition specialist, Dr. Mitchell earned her Ph.D. from the University of Tennessee and taught nutrition and health science at the University of Central Florida for over eight years. In addition to being the nutrition expert for ThirdAge.com, she is the coauthor of two books, *I'd Kill for a Cookie* and *Eat to Stay Young,* and is a contributing author to Macmillan Reference USA's *Guide to World Nutrition and Health.*

How to Contact:

Web site: www.susanmitchell.org
E-mail: drmitchell@fatisnotyourfate.com

DR. CATHERINE CHRISTIE is the director of the Nutrition Program and MSH Dietetic Internship at the University of North Florida. A registered dietitian, certified nutrition specialist, and fellow of the American Dietetic Association, she served for seven years as chairman of the Florida Dietetics and Nutrition Council, which regulates the nutrition profession. Dr. Christie currently serves as president-elect of the Florida Dietetic Association. She has been quoted in *USA Today, Family Circle, Reader's Digest, Women's Day,* and numerous other publications. She is the editor of the *Florida Manual of Medical Nutrition Therapy* and coeditor of Macmillan Reference USA's *Guide to World Nutrition and Health.* Dr. Christie is the coauthor of *I'd Kill for a Cookie* and *Eat to Stay Young.*

How to Contact:

E-mail: drchristie@fatisnotyourfate.com